Also by Andreas Moritz

• • •

The Amazing Liver and Gallbladder Flush

Timeless Secrets of Health and Rejuvenation

Lifting the Veil of Duality

It's Time to Come Alive

Simple Steps to Total Health

Hear the Whispers, Live Your Dream (Dec. 2008)

Heart Disease No More!

Diabetes – No More!

Ending the AIDS Myth

Heal Yourself with Sunlight

Sacred Santémony & Ener-Chi Art

All of the above are available at **www.ener-chi.com**, **www.amazon.com**,
and other online or physical bookstores

Cancer
Is Not
A Disease!

It's A Survival Mechanism

*Discover Cancer's Hidden
Purpose, Heal its Root Causes,
And Be Healthier Than Ever*

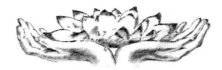

Your Health is in Your Hands

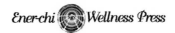

Ener-chi Wellness Press

ISBN-10: 097679442X
ISBN-13: 978-0976794424

Published by Ener-Chi Wellness Press—Ener-Chi.com, USA
Printed by Lightning Source Inc, USA

First edition, Cancer is not A Disease, October 2005
Second edition, Cancer is not A Disease, August 2008
Third edition (minor changes), Cancer is Not a Disease, February 2009

Cover Design and Artwork by Andreas Moritz
The picture on the cover is part of *Ener-Chi Art* (see http://www.ener-chi.com), designed to restore balanced Chi flow in all organs and systems of the body. This particular picture is designed to maintain proper Chi presence in the circulatory system/small intestines, an essential prerequisite for healing any cancer in the body.

Table of Contents:

This book is dedicated to those

who trust in the body's wisdom
and intelligence to heal itself;

—

who wish to work with the body,
and not against it;

—

who blame nobody for their illness
or misfortune, including themselves;

—

who perceive everything that happens to them
as useful, regardless how threatening or painful
it may appear to be;

—

and especially to those who are open and
prepared to be all of the above.

INTRODUCTION

What you are about to read may rock or even dismantle the very foundation of your beliefs about your body, health and healing. The title, "Cancer Is Not a Disease," may be unsettling for many, provocative to some, but encouraging for all. This book will serve as a revelation for those who are sufficiently open-minded to consider the possibility that cancer and other debilitating disorders are not actual diseases, but desperate and final attempts by the body to stay alive for as long as circumstances permit.

It will perhaps astound you to learn that a person who is afflicted with the main causes of cancer (which constitute the real illness) would most likely die quickly unless he actually grew cancer cells. In this work, I provide evidence to this effect.

I further claim that cancer will only occur after the body's main defense or healing mechanisms have already failed. In extreme circumstances, exposure to large amounts of cancer-producing agents (carcinogens) can bring about a collapse of the body's defenses within several weeks or months and allow for rapid and aggressive growth of a cancerous tumor. Usually, though, it takes many years, or even decades, for these so-called "malignant" tumors to form and become diagnostically noticeable.

Unfortunately, basic misconceptions or complete lack of knowledge about the reasons behind tumor growth have turned "misaligned" cancer cells into vicious monsters that have no other purpose but to kill us in retaliation for our sins or abusing the body. However, as you are about to find out, cancer is on our side, not against us. Unless we change our perception of what cancer really is, it will most likely resist treatment, particularly the most "advanced" and commonly applied methods. If you have cancer, and cancer is indeed part of the body's complex survival responses and not a disease, as I suggest it is, you must find answers to the following important questions:

- ❖ What reasons coerce your body into developing cancer cells?
- ❖ Once you have identified these reasons, will you be able to remove them?
- ❖ What determines the type and severity of cancer with which you are afflicted?
- ❖ If cancer is a survival mechanism, what needs to be done to prevent the body from taking recourse to such drastic measures of self-preservation?
- ❖ Since the body's original genetic design always favors the continuance of life and protection against adversities of any kind, why would the body permit self-destruction?
- ❖ Why do almost all cancers disappear by themselves, without medical intervention?
- ❖ Do radiation, chemotherapy and surgery actually cure cancer, or do cancer survivors heal due to other reasons, *in spite of* these radical, side-effect-loaded treatments?
- ❖ What roles do fear, frustration, low self-worth and repressed anger play in the origination and outcome of cancer?
- ❖ What is the spiritual growth lesson behind cancer?

To deal with the root causes of cancer, you must find satisfying and practical answers to the above questions. If you feel the inner urge to make sense of this life-changing event (cancer, that is), you will greatly benefit from continuing to read this book. Cancer can be your greatest opportunity to help restore balance to all aspects of your life, but it can also be the harbinger of severe trauma and suffering. Either way, you will discover that you are always in control of your body. To live in a human body, you must have access to a certain amount of life-sustaining energy. You may either use this inherent energy in a nourishing and self-sustaining way or in a destructive and debilitating way. In case you consciously or unconsciously choose negligence or self-abuse over loving attention and self-respect, your body will likely end up having to fight for its life. The main issue is not whether you have cancer but how you perceive it.

Cancer is but one of the many ways the body tries to change

the way you see and treat yourself, including your physical body. This inevitably brings up the subject of spiritual health, which plays at least as important a role in cancer as physical and emotional reasons do.

Cancer appears to be a highly confusing and unpredictable disorder. It seems to strike the very happy and the very sad, the rich and the poor, the smokers and the non-smokers, the very healthy and the not so healthy. People from all backgrounds and occupations can have cancer. However, if you dare look behind the mask of its physical symptoms, such as the type, appearance and behavior of cancer cells, you will find that cancer is not as coincidental or unpredictable as it seems to be.

What makes 50% of the American population so prone to developing cancer, when the other half has no risk at all? Blaming the genes for that is but an excuse to cover up ignorance of the real causes or lure people afflicted with cancer into costly treatment programs. Besides, any good genetic researcher would tell you that such a belief is void of any logic and outright unscientific.

Cancer has always been an extremely rare illness, except in industrialized nations during the past 40-50 years. Human genes have not significantly changed for thousands of years. Why would they change so drastically now, and suddenly decide to kill scores of people? The answer to this question, which I will further elaborate on in this book, is amazingly simple: Damaged or faulty genes do not kill anyone. Cancer does not kill a person afflicted with it! What kills a cancer patient is not the tumor, but the numerous reasons behind cell mutation and tumor growth. These root causes should be the focus of every cancer treatment, yet most oncologists typically ignore them. Constant conflicts, resentment, guilt and shame (known as stress), for example, can easily paralyze the body's most basic functions, and easily lead to the growth of a cancerous tumor.

After having seen thousands of cancer patients over a period of three decades, I began to recognize a certain pattern of thinking, believing and feeling that was common to most of them. To be more specific, I have yet to meet a cancer patient who does not feel burdened by some poor self-image, unresolved conflict and worries, or past emotional conflict/trauma that still lingers in his subconscious mind and cellular memories. Cancer, the physical disease, cannot occur unless there is a strong undercurrent of emotional uneasiness and deep-seated frustration.

Cancer patients typically suffer from lack of self-respect or worthiness, and often have what I call an "unfinished business" in their life. Cancer can actually be a way of revealing the source of such an unresolved, inner conflict. Furthermore, cancer can help them come to terms with such a conflict, and even heal it altogether. The way to take out weeds is to pull them out along with their roots. This is how we must treat cancer; otherwise, it may recur eventually.

The first chapter of this book provides you with profound insights into what cancer really is and stands for, seen from a physical perspective. It is an understanding of cancer you may never have come across before. This new and yet timeless comprehension of cancer allows for new approaches targeted at actually healing the causes of cancer instead of merely fixing its symptomatic manifestations.

Chapters Two and Three deal with the physical and emotional/spiritual causes, respectively. For clarities sake, I have tried to separate these categories, although I am very much aware that such a division is arbitrary and non-existent. I have done this for one purpose only: to emphasize that healing the causes of cancer must include restoring one's physical, emotional and spiritual wellbeing. Leaving out just one of these factors would undermine the chances of full recovery and eventually lead to the recurrence of cancer (most medically treated cancers reoccur). At least, such an incomplete approach would seriously affect one's mental and physical health and, foremost of all, one's state of happiness.

The following statement, which runs like a red thread through the entire book, is very important in the consideration of cancer: **"Cancer does not cause a person to be sick; it is the sickness of the person that causes the cancer."** To treat cancer successfully requires the patient to become whole again on all levels of his body, mind and spirit. Once the cancer causes have been properly identified, it will become apparent what needs to be done to achieve complete recovery. This is the subject matter of Chapter Four.

It is a medical fact that every person has cancer cells in the body at all times in his life. These cancer cells remain undetectable through standard tests until they have multiplied to several billion. When doctors announce to their cancer patients that the treatments they prescribed had successfully eliminated all cancer cells, they merely refer to tests that are able to identify the detectable size of cancer tumors. Standard cancer treatments may lower the number of cancer cells to an undetectable level, but this certainly cannot eradicate all cancer cells. As long as the causes of tumor growth remain intact, cancer may redevelop at any time and at any speed.

Curing cancer has little to do with getting rid of a group of detectable cancer cells. Treatments like chemotherapy and radiation are certainly capable of poisoning or burning many cancer cells, but they also destroy healthy cells in the bone marrow, gastrointestinal tract, liver, kidneys, heart, lungs, etc., which often leads to permanent irreparable damage of entire organs and systems in the body. The poisons of chemotherapy drugs alone cause such severe inflammation in every cell of the body that even the hair follicles can no longer hold on to the strands of hair. A real cure of cancer does not occur at the expense of destroying other vital parts of the body. It is achievable only when the causes of excessive growth of cancer cells have been removed or stopped. This book is dedicated to dealing with the causes of cancer, not with its symptoms. Treating cancer as if it were a disease is a trap that millions of people have fallen into and they have paid a high price for not attending to its root causes.

Chapter One

Cancer Is Not a Disease

Power in the Word

Cancer is the second leading cause of death for Americans. According to the American Cancer Society, about 1.2 million people will be diagnosed with cancer in the U.S. this year. More than 552,000 Americans will die of it. Among men, the top three cancer diagnoses are expected to be prostate cancer (180,400 cases), lung cancer (89,500 cases), and colorectal cancer (63,600 cases). The leading types of cancer among women are breast cancer (182,800 cases), lung cancer (74,600 cases), and colorectal cancer (66,600 cases).

In addition, there are tens of thousands of underprivileged people who have cancer, but will not even receive a diagnosis because they cannot afford health insurance or a visit to the doctor.

Cancer is not just a word, but also a statement that refers to abnormal or unusual behavior of the body's cells. However, in quite a different context, cancer is referred to as a star sign. When someone says you are a "cancer," are you going tremble with fear of dying? **Such a reaction is unlikely, because your interpretation of being of the cancer sign does not imply that you *have* cancer, the illness.** But if your doctor called you into his office and told you that you had cancer, you would most likely feel paralyzed, numb, terrified, hopeless, or all of the above. The word "cancer" has the potential to play a very disturbing and precarious role in your life, one that is capable of delivering a death sentence. Although being a cancer patient seems to start with the diagnosis of cancer, its causes may have been present for many years prior to the patient feeling ill. Within a brief moment, the word "cancer" can turn someone's entire world upside down.

1

Who or what in this world has bestowed this simple word or statement with such great power that it can preside over life and death? Or does it really possess this power? Could it actually be that our collective, social conviction that cancer is a killer disease, in addition to the aggressive treatments that follow diagnosis, are largely responsible for the current dramatic escalation of cancer in the Western hemisphere? Such a thought is too far fetched, you might say! In this book, however, I will make the point that cancer can have no power or control over you, unless you allow it to grow in response to the beliefs, perceptions, attitudes, thoughts, and feelings you have, as well as the life choices you make.

Would you be as afraid of cancer if you knew what caused it or at least understood what its underlying purpose was? Unlikely so! If the truth were told, you would probably do everything you could to remove the causes of the cancer and thereby create the preconditions for the body to heal itself.

A little knowledge—which is what you may call ignorance—is, in fact, a dangerous thing. Almost everyone, at least in the industrialized world, knows that drinking water from a filthy pond or polluted lake can cause life-threatening diarrhea. Yet, relatively few people realize that holding on to resentment, anger, and fear, avoiding exposure to the sun, not getting enough sleep, or eating junk foods, chemical additives, and artificial sweeteners is no less dangerous than drinking polluted water; these habits of life may just take a little longer to kill a person than tiny amoeba do.

Mistaken Judgment

We all know that if the foundation of a house is strong, the house can easily withstand external challenges, such as a violent storm. As we will see, cancer is merely an indication that something is missing in our body and in our life. Cancer shows that our physical, mental and spiritual life as a whole stands on shaky ground and is quite fragile, to say the least.

It would be foolish for a gardener to water the withering

leaves of a tree when he knows very well that the real problem is not where it appears to be, namely, on the level of those withered leaves. The dehydration of the leaves is merely a symptom of lacking water in the less apparent parts of the plant – its root system. By watering the roots of the plant, the gardener naturally attends to the causative level, and consequently, the whole plant becomes revived and resumes its normal growth. To the trained eye of a gardener, the symptom of withering leaves is not a dreadful disease. He recognizes that the dehydrated state of these leaves is but a direct consequence of withdrawn nourishment that they need to sustain themselves and the rest of the plant.

Although this example from nature may appear to be a simplistic analogy, it offers a profound understanding of some very complex disease processes in the human body. It accurately describes one of the most powerful and fundamental principles controlling all life forms on the planet. However skilled we may have become at manipulating the functions of our body through the tools of allopathic medicine, this basic law of nature cannot be suppressed or violated without paying the hefty price of side-effect-riddled suffering and pain on the physical, emotional, and spiritual levels.

I fervently challenge the statement that cancer is a killer disease. Furthermore, I will demonstrate that cancer is not a disease at all. Many people who received a "terminal" cancer sentence actually defied the prognosis and experienced complete remission. George, my first kidney cancer patient was one of them. His doctors at one of the most prestigious university hospitals in Germany had just "given" him three more weeks to live when he sought me out for help. According to them, his cancer was too advanced and widespread to consider having treatments of chemotherapy or radiation.

Healing Cancer Versus Fighting It

George had lost one of his kidneys to cancer one year earlier. After emerging from the operating room, his doctors gave him a "clean bill of health." They used the famous "we got it all" expression, which made a lot of sense to George; after all, they had removed the tumor, along with the entire kidney. Nevertheless, several months later his second kidney also started filling up with cancer, and the only "reasonable" advice they had for him was to take care of his personal affairs.

Fortunately for George, he didn't die. In total defiance of the death sentence that his doctors had given him, George felt that there should be something else he could do to at least extend his life by a few months. Within a mere three weeks of dealing with the causes of his illness, the cancer receded to a tiny speck, and during his next major check-up at the German cancer clinic six months later, was nowhere to be found. Fifteen years later, George still enjoys a state of perfect health, with no indication of a malfunctioning kidney.

I had given George neither a diagnosis nor a prognosis. What would have been the point of telling him how bad and hopeless his situation was? Besides, a doctor's "objective" statement that his patient's cancer is terminal (leading to his death) is actually a purely subjective viewpoint of a highly unpredictable situation. The doctor ties his so convincing and final judgment largely to past observations he has made with previous patients who suffered from similar symptoms. All this judgment does, however, is rule out the chance of recovery as a result of undergoing alternative treatments unknown to the treating physician. Just because the relatively young Western system of medicine does not know how to treat cancer successfully, does not imply that the ancient forms of medicine are helpless, too.

In orthodox medicine, patients are not encouraged to expect a spontaneous remission of their cancer. Doctors want to avoid giving them "false" hope, if there can be such a thing as false hope. Either there is hope or there is none, but hope cannot be wrong or false. The future is not written in stone. Nobody in this world can predict with complete certainty what is going to happen in the near or distant future. One may come up with a good guess of what the most likely probabilities might be, but none of these carry the stamp of absolute certainty. A young man with an extremely rare and inoperable large brain tumor, whose story was recently documented on prime time live television in the U.S., defied the prognosis of a very short life and continues to live quite actively and healthily several years afterward. He even got married recently.

To avoid the complications that arise from diagnosing diseases, such as making a person believe he is a helpless victim of some sort, I merely encouraged and motivated George to attend to the various factors responsible for causing and promoting cancer growth in the first place. Subsequently, his body naturally started to take care of the details, which included removing the symptom, cancer, in this case—a rather minor feat once the causes of the cancer were no longer present.

The total remission of George's cancer was neither the result of curing what appeared to be a horrible, self-perpetuating disease, nor was it a miracle. It was a simple process of giving back to the body what it needed to return to its most natural and normal state of balance. George merely ended the reasons why his body needed to fight for its life. As simple as it sounds, he healed himself by taking responsibility for all aspects of his life, including his body. The lesson that can be learned from George's experience is that true healing requires you to stop fighting; for fighting, as we shall see, is what actually prevents a true cure.

Searching for Answers

There is no cancer that has not been survived by someone, regardless of how far advanced it was. If even one person has succeeded in healing his cancer, there must be a mechanism for it, just as there is a mechanism for creating cancer. Every person on the planet has the capacity to do both. If you have been diagnosed with cancer, you may not be able to change the diagnosis, but it is certainly in your power to alter the destructive consequences that it (the diagnosis) may have on you, just as George did. The way you perceive the cancer and the steps you choose to take following the diagnosis are some of the most powerful determinants of your future wellness, or the lack of it. (Please also see Chapter Three, "Demystifying Cancer.")

The indiscriminate reference to "cancer" as a killer disease by professionals and lay people alike has turned cancer into a disorder with tragic consequences for the majority of today's cancer patients and their families. Cancer has become synonymous with extraordinary suffering, pain, and death. This perception continues despite the fact that 90-95 percent of all cancers appear and disappear of their own accord. Not a day passes without the body making millions of cancer cells. Some people, under severe temporary stress, make more cancer cells than usual and form clusters of cancerous cells that disappear again once they feel better. According to medical research, secretions of the DNA's powerful anticancer drug, *Interleukin II*, drop under physical and mental duress and increase again when the person becomes relaxed and joyful. Low secretions of Interleukin II increase the incidence of cancer in the body. However, people are generally not under severe stress all the time. Therefore, most cancers vanish without any form of medical intervention and without causing any real harm. **Right at this moment, millions of people are walking around with cancers in their body without having a clue that they have them. Likewise, millions of people heal their cancers without even knowing it.** Overall, there are many more spontaneous remissions of cancer than there are diagnosed and treated cancers.

The truth is, relatively few cancers actually become "terminal" or are even detected. The vast majority of cancers remain undiagnosed and are not found until autopsy. Typically, these people don't die because of cancer. They don't even have symptoms that could prompt the doctor to prescribe any of the standard cancer-detecting tests. It should raise everyone's eyebrows that 30 - 40 times as many cases of thyroid, pancreatic, and prostate cancer are found in autopsy than are detected by doctors. The British medical journal Lancet published a study in 1993 that showed early screening often leads to unnecessary treatment. The reason for that? Although 33 percent of autopsies reveal prostate cancer, only 1 percent die from it. After age 75, half of males may have prostate cancer, but only 2 percent die from it. New official recommendations (August 2008) call for oncologists to no longer treat men with prostate cancer past the age of 75 years because the treatments do more harm than good and offer no advantages over no treatment at all.

It must be noted that these low mortality rates only apply to those who have neither been diagnosed with cancer nor received any treatment for cancer. Mortality rates, however, increase drastically if cancers are being diagnosed and treated, which clearly shows what does the killing. Once diagnosed, the vast majority of cancers are never given a chance to disappear on their own. They are promptly targeted with an arsenal of deadly weapons such as chemotherapy drugs, radiation, and the surgical knife. "Sleeping" tumors that would never really cause much harm to the body, may now be aroused into powerful defensive reactions and become aggressive, not unlike relatively harmless bacteria that turn into dangerous superbugs when attacked by antibiotic medication. It makes absolutely no sense that at a time you need to strengthen the body's most important healing system—the immune system—you would subject yourself to radical treatments that actually weaken or destroy the immune system.

The problem with cancer patients is that, terrified by the diagnosis, they submit their bodies to these cutting/burning/poisoning procedures that, more likely than not, will lead them more rapidly to the day of final sentencing: "We have to tell you with our deepest regret that there is nothing more that can be done to help you."

The most pressing question is not, "How advanced or dangerous is my cancer?" but, "What am I doing or not doing that puts my body into a situation of having to fight for its life?" Why do some people go through cancer as if it were the flu? Are they just lucky, or is there a mechanism at work that triggers the healing? On the contrary, what is the hidden element that prevents the body from healing cancer naturally, that makes cancer so dangerous, if indeed it is dangerous at all?

The answers to all these queries lie with the person who has the cancer, and does not depend on the degree of a particular cancer's "viciousness" or the advanced stage to which it appears to have progressed. Do you believe that cancer is a disease? You will most likely answer, "Yes," given the "informed" opinion that the medical industry and mass media have fed to the masses for many decades. Yet, the more important but rarely asked question remains, "Why do you think cancer is a disease?" You may answer, "Because I know cancer kills people every day." I would then question you further, "How do you know that it is the cancer that kills people?" You would probably argue that most people who have cancer die, so obviously it must be the cancer that kills them. Besides, you may reason, all the expert doctors tell us so.

Let me ask you another question, a rather strange one: "How do you know for sure that you are the daughter/son of your father and not of another man?" Is it because your mother told you so? What makes you think that your mother told you the truth? Probably because you believe her; and you have no reason not to. After all, she is your mother, and mothers do not lie about these things. Or do they? Although you will never really know with absolute certainty that the person you believe to be your father is, in fact, your father, you nevertheless have turned what you subjectively believe into something that you "know," into an irrefutable truth.

Although no scientific proof whatsoever exists to show that cancer is a disease (versus a healing attempt), most people will insist that it is a disease because this is what they have been told to believe. Yet this belief is only hearsay based on other people's opinions. These other people heard the same "truth" from someone else. Eventually, the infallible doctrine that cancer is a disease can be traced to some doctors who expressed their subjective feelings or beliefs about what they had observed and published them in some review articles or medical reports. Other doctors agreed with their opinion, and before long, it became a "well-established fact" that cancer is a vicious illness that somehow gets hold of people in order to kill them. However, the truth of the matter may actually be quite different and more rational and scientific than that.

The Gene/Cancer Myth

Extensive scientific research conducted in the field of cellular biology over the past 10 years has already proved that genes do not cause disease, but are, in fact, influenced and altered by changes in the environment, from the very first moments in the mother's womb to the last moments in a person's adult life. Cellular biologists now recognize that the conditions and occurrences in the external surroundings and internal physiology, and more importantly, our *perception* of the environment, directly control the activity of our genes.

Along these lines, one type of gene that plays a role in normal cell growth, an *oncogene,* can be altered by its environment, the cell's internal terrain and surroundings, to contribute to the uncontrolled growth of a tumor. Oncogenes affect the way cells use energy and multiply. For example, in some cancers, the *ras gene* (an oncogene) mutates, and produces a protein that stimulates cells to divide prematurely. It is important to understand that genes do not mutate because they become "bored" with being "normal" or because they want to become malignant. Rather, they are left with no other choice but to mutate, which allows them to survive a hostile, toxic "tumor milieu" that has been created by factors other than genetic ones. A tumor-milieu, a cell environment that is poorly oxygenated and highly acidic, is the ideal medium to favor the growth of cancer cells and the microorganisms found in cancerous tumors.

As difficult as this may be to come to terms with, defective genes cannot be the cause of cancer. It is a fact that millions of people with defective genes will never develop the diseases these defects are supposed to cause. You can actually remove the nucleus of a cancer cell, and yet for several weeks or months the cell will continue to live and behave in exactly the same abnormal way as before. "Silencing" is the word used to describe a process by which environment and behavior regulate gene expression and environmental switches activate cancer. Genes comprise a complex blueprint that is constantly adapting to external changes or influences.

Genetic blueprints are not capable of causing or perpetuating diseases. If they were, the cell would malfunction or die as soon as you removed the genes, which are contained in the nucleus, from the cell. To repeat, a healthy cell continues to live perfectly normally for weeks on end, even if the genes are not present.

Your DNA's only activity is to make a copy (RNA) of itself and to use this copy (of the genetic codes) to produce the many different proteins needed for the numerous functions and processes in the body. To understand what cancer really is, we have to understand this important fact: The blueprint (genetic code of the cell) changes in an abnormal way *only* when the information delivered to the cell via its external environment invokes a continuous stress response within the cell. What does this mean in practical terms?

Each cell in the body is capable of producing adrenaline and other stress hormones, and it does so when you experience an external or internal threat that requires a "fight or flight" response. The threat could consist of any number of influences, such as food additives like Aspartame and MSG; an antibiotic or steroid drug; crossing a busy highway; the fear of facing an angry spouse or authority figure; or a profound sense of insecurity.

Under the influence of the secreted stress hormones, normal cell functions are undermined. In fact, the genetic blueprint (DNA) receives distorted information that, in turn, alters the cell's genetic behavior. Consequently, the DNA's production of natural chemicals, such as the anti-cancer drug *Interleukin II* and the anti-viral drug *Interferon,* begins to drop instantly and significantly. The cell's health and defensive capabilities are seriously compromised if the threat or stress persists over a period longer than just a few minutes or hours. (This kind of stress is a daily reality for millions of people in today's world.) Cells cannot fulfill their normal responsibilities when "under siege" for days, months, or even years.

Allopathic medicine has a name for this normal response by cells under prolonged stress: "chronic disease."

When the body ingests a harmful medical drug (all drugs contain poisons and are, therefore, injurious to the cells), or is exposed to such stressors as constant negative thoughts, feelings, emotions, or behaviors, insufficient nourishment, inadequate amounts of sleep, lack of sun exposure, dehydration, or toxins, this will alter the behavior of *all* its 60-100 trillion cells. Cancer occurs when cellular balance is threatened and the cell has to take recourse to more extreme measures of defending or protecting itself. The weakest cells are affected first. Genetic mutation from a normal cell to a cancer cell is merely a normal survival response to a threat that prevents the cell from doing its job according to the body's original genetic blueprint.

The possibility that cancer is a survival mechanism has never been considered in the past and is not part of the cancer discussion today. This has had and still has, to this day, fatal consequences.

Not too long ago, expert scientists believed that the Earth was flat and stationary. After all, they saw with their own eyes that the sun "fell off" the horizon every evening and "rose" again every morning, although on the opposite side. This indisputable "truth" was difficult to root out because it was a phenomenon that the masses witnessed each and every day. They knew well that the entire natural world depended on sunrise and sunset, the cycles of day and night. Little did they realize that what their eyes saw so clearly was not what was actually occurring.

Today, we only smile at such a notion of ignorance. Yet, with modern diseases and cancer, specifically, we are living by the same old myths handed down to us from generation to generation. Are we not also falling into the trap of blindly believing what other people have accepted as their subjective, personal truth? "But today it is different," you may argue, "because we have objective, verifiable scientific research to prove what is real and what is not." I may have to disappoint you here.

First, almost all scientific research studies are actually based on the subjective ideas, feelings, and thoughts of the scientist conducting the experiment. Second, the research is subjected to an almost infinite number of possible and often highly variable influences that can alter the outcome of the experiment in several unpredictable ways. Third, science rarely finds anything that it did not expect to find. Researchers tend to research something they subjectively feel is worth investigating. The purpose of their research is merely to fulfill the expectations they already have about the outcome of the experiment. If you are looking for something you subjectively expect to be true, you are likely to find objective proof for your assumption.

When genetic scientists proposed that genes control the body and behavior, they developed the *Human Genome* project to prove exactly that hypothesis. Paid for by the pharmaceutical companies, these scientists had just one major objective: they had to fulfill the expectations of the big pharma conglomerate to patent genes for new, expensive "breakthrough" treatments that generate vast amounts of wealth. Nowhere do they mention the proven biomedical fact that genes do not control anything. The genes' only function and purpose are to reproduce cells. How genes do that largely depends on you and what you expose yourself to. In fact, all genes in your body are controlled by the cells' environment and its influences, including your personal perceptions and beliefs.

Dismal Success of Anti-Cancer Treatments

Just take the placebo effect[1] as an example. A placebo (which literally means, "I shall please") is included as an indispensable element of every scientific study conducted today. The placebo effect is purely based on the subjective feelings of a person. Each person who is tested for the efficacy of a medical drug believes in the drug in a unique and unpredictable way. A certain number of people may have a hopeful, trusting disposition and, therefore, a stronger placebo response than others. Others may be suffering from depression, which is known to affect a person's ability to respond positively to any kind of treatment. As a result, one study may "prove" a particular drug to be effective for, let us say, a certain kind of cancer. However, if a repeat experiment is conducted with different subjects, this drug may turn out to be ineffective when compared to the placebo response. For this reason, pharmaceutical companies instruct their paid researchers

---

[1] A placebo is a term that describes the administration of a sugar pill or dummy procedure in order to test whether a drug or procedure is more effective than the power of belief. In an article in the *Guardian* (Thursday, June 20, 2002), Jerome Burne reported that "new research suggests that placebos work surprisingly well, in fact, rather better than some conventional drugs."

to publish *only* the most favorable findings from these various experiments. Those parts of the study where the drug has had no or only an insignificant advantage over the placebo effect are simply omitted from the study's final report.

The drug companies reporting their findings to the Food and Drug Administration (FDA) only need to prove that the tested drug has shown some benefit in some people. If the researchers manage to recruit enough candidates with a positive disposition that are likely to produce a good placebo response to the drug treatment, they may hit the jackpot and produce a "convincing" study, and a marketable drug. This is a no-brainer for drug makers since FDA approval is granted to anti-cancer drugs based on response rates that are at best in the 10-20 percent range (as happened, for example, with the popular drugs, Avastin, Erbitux, and Iressa). In addition, the "success" of most clinical cancer studies is measured by tumor shrinkage instead of mortality rate. In other words, even if most of the subjects died but had their tumors shrunk through aggressive treatments, the study would be hailed as a great success and a medical breakthrough.

Any such attempt to treat the human body as if it were a machine that just responds to mechanical or chemical manipulation is bound to have serious setbacks. Such an approach is not only unscientific, but also unethical and potentially harmful. For many cancer patients whose immune systems are already compromised, just one dose of chemotherapy or radiation can turn out to be fatal.

Senior cancer physician, Dr. Charles Moertel of the famous Mayo Clinic in Rochester, Minnesota, once aptly summarized the modern cancer treatment dilemma in the following words: **"Our most effective regimens are fraught with risks and side effects and practical problems, and after this price is paid by all the patients we have treated, only a small fraction are rewarded with a transient period of usually incomplete tumor regression."**

The success record of modern cancer therapy is dismal, significantly less than even the weakest placebo response. On the average, remission occurs in only about 7% of cancer patients. Moreover, there is no evidence that this discouragingly low 7%

"success rate" results from the treatments offered; it could just as well be in spite of the treatments. This is more likely, since not treating cancer at all has a much higher success rate than treating it. A drug treatment that promises temporary tumor shrinkage in 10% of patients is not a promising therapy; rather, it is a dangerous gamble with their life.

Statistical Fraud

The cancer industry tries to use statistical "evidence" to convince you that you need to entrust your life into their hands. However, any chemotherapy success stories are limited to relatively obscure types of cancer, such as *Burkitt's lymphoma* and *choriocarcinoma,* so rare that many clinicians have never seen a single case. Childhood leukemia constitutes less than 2 percent of all cancers, and thus hardly influences the overall success rate. Chemo's supposedly strong track record with Hodgkin's disease (lymphoma) is a blunt lie. Children who are successfully treated for Hodgkin's disease are 18 times more likely to develop secondary malignant tumors later in life (*New England Journal of Medicine*, March 21, 1996). According to the National Cancer Institute (*NCI Journal* 87:10), patients who underwent chemotherapy were 14 times more likely to develop leukemia and 6 times more likely to develop cancers of the bones, joints, and soft tissues than those patients who did not undergo chemotherapy. Yet if you have a child with lymphoma and refuse treatment for the above well-documented reasons, you face prosecution by the law, and your child may be taken away from you. The bottom line is this: Although only 2-4% of cancers respond to chemotherapy, it has now become standard procedure to prescribe chemo drugs for most cancers. The percentage of people with cancer in the U.S. who receive chemotherapy is 75%.

In its cancer investigations, the *U.S. General Accounting Office* (GAO) reported: "For the majority of the cancers we examined, the actual improvements (in survival) have been small or have been overestimated by the published rates... It is difficult to find that there has been much progress...(For breast cancer), there is a slight improvement...(which) is considerably less than reported."

One cancer researcher said it even more bluntly: "The five year cancer survival statistics of the American Cancer Society are very misleading. They now count things that are not cancer, and, because we are able to diagnose at an earlier stage of the disease, patients falsely appear to live longer. Our whole cancer research in the past 20 years has been a failure. More people over 30 are dying from cancer than ever before... More women with mild or benign diseases are being included in statistics and reported as being 'cured'. When government officials point to survival figures and say they are winning the war against cancer they are using those survival rates improperly." ~ Dr. J. Bailer (*New England Journal of Medicine,* Sept/Oct 1990.)

Official cancer statistics simply omit African Americans, a group that actually has the highest incidence of cancers. They also don't include patients with lung cancer which is the most common cause of cancer-related death in men and the second most common in women. However, the statistical data include millions of people with diseases that are not life-threatening and are easily curable, such as localized cancers of the cervix, non-spreading cancers, skin cancers and *ductal carcinoma in situ* or DCIS—the most common kind of non-invasive breast cancer. Even pre-cancers are included to boost the dismal success rate of modern cancer therapy. Most pre-cancers never develop into cancer.

With a death rate that is not lower, but is actually 6% higher, in 1997 than in 1970, there is nothing to suggest that modern cancer therapy is scientific, effective, or worth the pain, effort, and vast expenditures. This trend has continued to this day. With a failure rate of at least 93%, medical cancer therapy cannot be considered a treatment at all, but rather a serious threat to societal health. Albert Braverman M.D., sums up the vicious cycle perpetuated by the currently used medical model: "Many medical oncologists recommend chemotherapy for virtually any tumor, with a hopefulness undiscouraged by almost invariable failure." ~ *1991 Lancet, "Medical Oncology in the 90s."*

The Power of Belief

According to the laws of quantum physics, in any scientific experiment the observer (a researcher) influences and alters the object of observation on a very fundamental level (observer-observed relationship). This fundamental principle of physics applies to you just as much. After all, your body is composed of molecules that are made of atoms; these atoms are composed of subatomic particles, which in turn, are made of energy and information. There is actually not even a trace of matter in what we consider physical creation. Although something may appear to be as solid and concrete as a rock, there is nothing solid about it; only your sensory perception makes it appear so.

Your thoughts also are merely forms of energy and information that influence other forms of energy and information, including the cells of your body. For example, if you are sad about something that happened to you, your body posture changes and your eyes lose their luster. Eye cells, like all other cells in the body, respond to your thoughts as a soldier follows the orders of his superior. The bottom line is this: **If you believe strongly enough that you have cancer or if you are afraid of it, you face a significant risk of manifesting it in your body.**

The placebo effect can work both ways. The belief that you have a deadly disease can be just as powerful as the belief that a certain medical drug can heal you. In an instant, the energy of your thoughts and beliefs delivers the information they contain to every cell in your body. The energy and information that make up the atoms, molecules, genes, cells, organs and systems in your body have no agenda of their own. They are certainly not malicious. All they do is follow orders. You manifest both what you like and what you do not like. In other words, you are what you believe. Furthermore, what you believe is determined by the way you see or perceive things. Clearly, your interpretation of cancer as a disease will likely turn it into a disease *for you*. Otherwise, cancer would just be a survival mechanism or a signal for you to take care of those aspects of your life that you have neglected thus far.

If you believe that cancer is a disease, you are more likely to be inclined to fight against it, physically, emotionally, and spiritually. If you are strong-willed and the weapons you are using are powerful, you may be able to subdue this "enemy" of yours, at least for a while. In such a case, you will be proud of having "beaten" the cancer and, perhaps, you will praise the doctors or the medical treatment you endured for having saved your life. If you are weak and you use these same weapons in an attempt to destroy the cancer, you are likely going to succumb to what you would consider a malicious enemy. The doctor will express with regret that your body did not sufficiently "respond" to the treatment (the weapons), claiming that he tried everything and that nothing more could be done. He will neglect to inform you that the weapons he has put into your body can be deadly.

Chemotherapy is so poisonous that leaking a few drops of the drug onto your hand can severely burn it. If drops fall on a concrete floor, they can burn holes into it. Spilling any chemo-therapeutic drug in the hospital or anywhere en route is classified as a major biohazard and it requires specialists with space-suits to dispose of it.

Just imagine the holes chemotherapy creates inside your blood vessels, lymphatic ducts, and organ tissues when you undergo infusion after infusion! I have looked at the irises of patients (using iridology) who have gone through chemotherapy, and I saw the considerable erosion and damage of tissues throughout the body. Yes, this drug destroys cancer cells, but along with them, many of your healthy cells, too. Your entire body becomes inflamed. For this reason, your hair falls out when you undergo chemotherapy or radiation, and you cannot digest food anymore. Many patients develop anorexia – the loss of appetite or desire to eat. But this is not the only risk you can expect from modern cancer therapies. "Chemotherapy and radiation can increase the risk of developing a second cancer by up to 100 times," according to Dr. Samuel S. Epstein ~ *Congressional Record, Sept. 9, 1987.*

Given the extreme suffering cancer patients are being subjected to by undergoing cancer treatments, people like Jackie Onassis were fortunate to have died quickly, although unnecessarily. Tim O'Shea wrote in *To The Cancer Patient*: "...Chemo drugs are some of the most toxic substances ever designed to go into a human body, their effects are very serious, and are often the direct cause of death. Like the case of Jackie Onassis, who underwent chemo for one of the rare diseases in which it generally has some beneficial results: non-Hodgkins lymphoma. She went into the hospital on Friday and was dead by Tuesday."

I have personally seen cancer patients who successfully and naturally reversed their cancers but were then talked into taking a round of chemotherapy just to be sure to "get it all." They all died within a day or two of the first treatment.

The methods of modern medicine don't fight disease, they fight the body. Disease is the body's way of healing itself, and modern treatment is a sure way to impair or even destroy this ability.

Creating a Monster Where There Is None

All this raises a very important question: could it possibly be that cancer is not a disease, but a survival mechanism of the body designed to remove something that does not belong there? If so, would it not make more sense to support the body in its natural drive to remove such obstructions rather than to suppress its effort with aggressive, destructive means? Most intelligent people would agree with this. For when the obstruction is gone, there would be no further need for the body to continue relying on such a desperate survival mechanism as cancer.

An old saying goes, "The proof of the pudding lies in the eating." You will not know how the pudding tastes until you eat it. If you remove the causes of an illness and the illness disappears by itself, you will know for certain that there was no illness in the first place. There were only reasons that made the body do things it normally would not do. Whenever you prevent the body from conducting its normal activities, it has no other choice than to apply corrective measures that can at least alleviate the situation and restore some of its basic functions.

Most people in the Western hemisphere, though, have not had

the opportunity to go through the learning experience of self-empowerment that can result from supporting the body while experiencing an illness, rather than fighting against it. If they fall ill, they immediately believe the body must be doing something wrong, whereas in reality it is doing something right to rectify a difficult situation they have created or allowed for whatever known or unknown reason. If they hold onto the belief, "The body is making me sick," long enough, that misinterpretation of the real situation will turn into something that they eventually experience to be true.

Furthermore, if many other people believe the same thing, it becomes an established "fact" we have to live with. Before long, an entire population knows this "fact" and behaves accordingly, with fear and apprehension. Their truth becomes a self-fulfilling prophecy, and natural instincts and common sense are thrown out of the window.

Collectively, we have created an atmosphere that expects disease. Most people in the Western world turn to a doctor for every little problem they have. Even during pregnancy, the battery of checkups a woman and her growing fetus must undergo, program the mother and child for a life-long dependency upon doctors. Now we must have a doctor for the delivery (although billions of healthy babies have successfully been delivered without one). We also need a doctor to administer the various childhood vaccinations (another cause of cancer), to prescribe antibiotics for an ear or throat infection, to tell us whether we need to take out the tonsils or appendix, and to prescribe drugs for nervousness and attention deficit disorder because we live on sugar, food additives, and fast foods or are deprived of our parents' loving and caring attention. Furthermore, a doctor is needed to tell us that we need statin drugs for an elevated cholesterol level, diuretic pills for high blood pressure, and an angioplasty to unclog our blocked arteries. The list goes on almost indefinitely.

The masterminds of collective programming (those with the most vested interests in taking advantage of the ignorance of the masses) have succeeded in manipulating the food and medical industries for their own profit and control. Today, the masses no longer think for themselves and have lost trust in their innate and instinctive healing ability. They turn to an industry that has no interest in keeping them healthy. Dr. Martin Shapiro, University of California, Los Angeles made this unsettling remark about the precarious situation we are finding ourselves confronted with: "Cancer researchers, medical journals, and the popular media all have contributed to a situation in which many people with common malignancies are being treated with drugs not known to be effective."

Many natural cures for cancer exist, more now than ever, but none of them are being researched, endorsed, or promoted by those who claim to be the health custodians of the nation. The American Cancer Society, the National Cancer Institute, the American Medical Association (AMA), the Food and Drug Administration (FDA), and the major oncology centers all feel threatened by the successes of alternative cancer therapies. Of course, this is not difficult to understand, given the high failure rate (93%) of medical therapies.

The world-renowned health researchers Robert Houston and Gary Null poignantly revealed the reasons behind the medical industry's cancer strategy: "A solution to cancer would mean the termination of research programs, the obsolescence of skills, the end of dreams of personal glory; triumph over cancer would dry up contributions to self-perpetuating charities... It would mortally threaten the present clinical establishments by rendering obsolete the expensive surgical, radiological and chemotherapeutic treatments in which so much money, training and equipment is invested... The new therapy must be disbelieved, denied, discouraged and disallowed at all costs, regardless of actual testing results, and preferably without any testing at all."

The prominent cancer researcher and professor at the University of California (Berkely and Davis), Dr. Hardin Jones, had this to say about the current cancer dilemma: "It is most likely that, in terms of life expectancy, the chance of survival is no better with than without treatment, and there is the possibility that treatment may make the survival time of cancer less." After analyzing cancer survival statistics for several decades, Dr. Jones, a professor at the University of California, concluded that

"...patients are as well, or better off untreated." Jones' disturbing assessment has never been refuted. Dr. Jones has been quoted as follows: "My studies have proven conclusively that cancer patients who refuse chemotherapy and radiation actually live up to four times longer than treated cases, including untreated breast cancer cases."

When not treating cancer brings about better results than treating it, the question arises, "Why then do our health agencies allow, encourage, and even enforce treatments that have been proven to kill cancer patients prematurely?" Perhaps the AMA has the answer to that question. One of the AMA's stated objectives and obligations is to protect the income of its members (medical doctors). The biggest income of AMA members is generated by treating cancer patients. On the average, every cancer patient is worth $50,000. If ever a cancer cure were officially recognized in this country (USA), it would threaten the income and livelihood of AMA members. The bylaws of the AMA practically prohibit the promotion of a cure for cancer.

After 60 years of intensive research and hundreds of billions spent on treatments for cancer that have killed thousands of patients, we are facing the collective challenge of our own survival. The only reasonable alternative to stop this fabricated monster is to learn the skills of healing ourselves. The other option will most likely bankrupt our countries, endanger our livelihoods, and lead us into the abyss of self-destruction.

Medical Predicaments

Every person with a sound medical background knows that the symptom of an illness is not the real illness, yet the majority of doctors today treat the symptoms as if they were the disease. Without knowing the causes of the vast majority of the over 40,000 listed diseases, medical textbooks and practitioners nevertheless speak of "effective treatments" for these diseases. The disease agencies that were originally set up to protect the population against false claims of cures insist that only medical drugs can "diagnose and cure diseases." Their agents seek out anyone who makes such claims using different methods than are being propagated by the medical industry and the drug cartels. Accordingly, anyone who says that a natural and harmless herb or food does the same or even better, violates the law and risks prosecution. That prescription drugs like Vioxx have killed and injured hundreds of thousands of people does not seem to encourage these agencies to go out and warn the masses to think twice about taking prescription drugs. This would give the nearly one million people who die each year from the devastating side effects caused by prescription drugs a chance to save their lives.

You always create harmful side effects when you treat the symptoms of disease without removing its underlying cause(s). How scientific or reasonable can it be to treat a disease for which the cause remains obscure? How much medical expertise can a prominent oncologist claim to have if he treats your cancer without having a clue where it is coming from or why it has occurred?

One of the key problems is that today's medical schools do not train their students to think for themselves when it comes to understanding the underlying causes of an illness. Medical doctors are required to follow a rigid protocol or treatment plan, and if they deviate from it, this could easily cost them their license to practice medicine. They may even end up in jail, like so many doctors who out of kindness and compassion have offered alternative, unauthorized treatments to their patients. Can we, therefore, reasonably expect to find out from the medical doctors and the technologies they employ, what really bothers us when we are sick? This is highly unlikely, although I am pleased to say there is a steadily increasing number of exceptions.

For the most part, we remain in the Dark Ages with regard to true healing. According to independent reports by the prestigious *New England Journal of Medicine*, a wing of the American Congress, and the World Health Organization (WHO), 85-90 percent of all medical procedures used by today's medical establishment are unproved and not backed up by scientific research. This includes almost every diagnostic procedure and treatment modality that is offered to you in your doctor's office or by your local hospital—most notably, the use of chemotherapy drugs and radiation.

If your car has engine trouble, would you entrust it to a mechanic who offered you a 10 percent guarantee of fixing it? I don't think so. You would more likely take your car to someone who is properly trained to look for and repair the causes of the malfunctioning engine rather than making a couple of superficial adjustments. Suffering from a disease means that there is something gone awry with the human "engine," if you will. Our medical practitioners, however, are not trained to deal with the root causes of chronic illness. Their training is dedicated instead to alleviating or shutting down the symptoms that indicate the body is trying to deal with an underlying imbalanced situation. Removing the symptoms actually suppresses the body's (and the mind's) attempt to deal with the real problem. The medical industry has brainwashed the masses to believe that their symptoms are actually diseases, and by suppressing or removing the symptoms, the diseases will vanish along with them.

If we cannot turn to medical doctors for true assistance and enlightenment in our quest for health and healing, could perhaps medical researchers bring us the answers we seek? This is just as unlikely. Most researchers are hired and sponsored by large drug corporations whose main interest lies in subduing and eliminating the symptoms of disease, not the disease itself. The main motivating force behind today's healthcare system, or shall I say, sickness care system, is the incessant need or greed to amass money, power, and control. The desire to help humanity to achieve health and vitality is shared only by those doctors and health practitioners who have genuine love and compassion for their fellow human beings.

The symptom-oriented approach to treating disease generates a tremendous number of potential symptomatic side effects that, in turn, require further treatment. Since none of the chosen treatment modalities are cause-oriented, there are bound to be continuously escalating complications in the future. This guarantees that there will always be enough patients who need medical attention and medical insurance. This trend, of course, will continue only for as long as the masses remain ignorant of their potential self-healing abilities.

As already mentioned, it is not in the best interest of the medical industry, including the pharmaceutical companies, to find a real cure for cancer or for any other chronic illnesses, for this would make the treatment of disease symptoms obsolete. Removing the cause(s) of an illness almost never requires a separate approach that deals with the symptoms of the illness, for these would disappear on their own once the underlying causes are addressed. Unless used for emergencies, costly methods of medical intervention, such as allopathic drugs, complex diagnostic procedures, radiation, and surgery are unnecessary. They also deceive patients and are potentially harmful to their health.[2]

At least 900,000 people die each year in the United States alone because of side effects caused by these symptom-suppressing, alleviating approaches. Since our present healthcare system promotes and encourages the treatment of symptoms of disease rather than the prevention of disease, it is one of the most clever and profitable investment schemes ever devised. The system lures unsuspecting people into having their symptoms treated, promising them relief while actually ensuring that the side effects from these treatments will almost certainly turn them into patients for life. The result is a permanent and ever-increasing source of income for drug companies, shareholders, medical institutions and medical practitioners.

If universal healthcare becomes a reality in the U.S., we will also experience a massive escalation of diseases and disease-related fatalities. Many people who currently cannot afford costly medical expenses or medical insurance tend to seek more natural, inexpensive ways of dealing with illness; or else they don't seek any treatment at all. Given the high fatality rate among people receiving medical treatment, the risk of dying from no treatment at all is actually very slim.[3] The no-treatment, low fatality risk, however, would be discouraged by "free healthcare." When I lived in Cyprus (Europe) in the 1980s I witnessed an entire population that used to rely mostly on natural methods of healing

---

[2] For details, see *Timeless Secrets of Health and Rejuvenation*.
[3] See the scientific evidence to that effect in Chapter 15, *What Doctors should be Telling You*, of *Timeless Secrets of Health and Rejuvenation*.

for thousands of years suddenly become hooked on the modern medical system because it became freely available. Giving something away for free has always been an effective marketing tactic to make people do or buy what they otherwise would never do or buy. Offering free healthcare has deceived and misleads the people of Cyprus, Germany, France, England, Canada, and it will do the same for the people of the United States, if implemented.

This is not to say that this trend is entirely the fault of the medical system. As long as people do not take responsibility for themselves, for their physical and emotional health, and for their dietary habits and lifestyle, we will have such a dangerous system in place. Millions of people experience devastating consequences resulting from medical treatments that are not warranted at all. Cancer patients, for example, tend to experience the most traumatic side effects because of the highly invasive nature of the treatments involved. The standard treatments for cancer are not meant to heal, but to destroy. The potential benefits of these treatments are not only questionable but also, according to one of the most comprehensive documented studies, non-existent. (See below.)

Can You Trust Chemotherapy?

Former White House press secretary Tony Snow died in July 2008 at the age of 53, following a series of chemotherapy treatments for colon cancer. In 2005, Snow had his colon removed and underwent six months of chemotherapy after being diagnosed with colon cancer. Two years later (2007), Snow underwent surgery to remove a growth in his abdominal area, near the site of the original cancer. "This is a very treatable condition," said Dr. Allyson Ocean, a gastrointestinal oncologist at Weill Cornell Medical College. "Many patients, because of the therapies we have, are able to work and live full lives with quality while they're being treated. Anyone who looks at this as a death sentence is wrong." But of course we now know, Dr. Ocean was dead wrong.

The media headlines proclaimed Snow died from colon

cancer, although they knew he didn't have a colon anymore. Apparently, the malignant cancer had "returned" (from where?) and "spread" to the liver and elsewhere in his body. In actual fact, the colon surgery severely restricted his normal eliminative functions, thereby overburdening the liver and tissue fluids with toxic waste. The previous series of chemo-treatments inflamed and irreversibly damaged a large number of cells in his body, and also impaired his immune system—a perfect recipe for growing new cancers. Now unable to heal the causes of the original cancer (in addition to the newly created ones), Snow's body developed new cancers in the liver and other parts of the body.

The mainstream media, of course, still insist Snow died from colon cancer, thus perpetuating the myth that it is only the cancer that kills people, not the treatment. Nobody seems to raise the important point that it is extremely difficult for a cancer patient to actually heal from this condition while being subjected to the systemic poisons of chemotherapy and deadly radiation. If you are bitten by a poisonous snake and don't get an antidote for it, isn't it likely that your body becomes overwhelmed by the poison and, therefore, cannot function anymore?

Before Tony Snow began his chemo-treatments for his second colon cancer, he still looked healthy and strong. But after a few weeks into his treatment, he started to develop a coarse voice, looked frail, turned gray and lost his hair. Did the cancer do this to him? Certainly not. Cancer doesn't do such a thing, but chemical poisoning does. He actually looked more ill than someone who has been bitten by a poisonous snake.

Do the mainstream media ever report about the overwhelming scientific evidence that shows chemotherapy has zero benefits in the 5-year survival rate of colon cancer patients?[4] Or how many oncologists stand up for their cancer patients and protect them against chemotherapy treatment which they know can cause them to die far more quickly than if they received no treatment at all?

---

[4] Confirmation of deficient mismatch repair (dMMR) as a predictive marker for lack of benefit from 5-FU based chemotherapy in stage II and III colon cancer (CC): a pooled molecular reanalysis of randomized chemotherapy trials. (D. J. Sargent, S. Marsoni, S. N. Thibodeau, et al.)

Can you trustingly place your life into their hands when you know that most of them would not even consider chemotherapy for themselves if they were diagnosed with cancer? What do they know that you don't? The news is spreading fast that in the United States physician-caused fatalities now exceed 750,000 each year. Perhaps, many doctors no longer trust in what they practice, for good reasons.

"Most cancer patients in this country die of chemotherapy... Chemotherapy does not eliminate breast, colon or lung cancers. This fact has been documented for over a decade. Yet doctors still use chemotherapy for these tumors... Women with breast cancer are likely to die faster with chemo than without it." — Alan Levin, M.D.

An investigation by the Department of Radiation Oncology, Northern Sydney Cancer Centre, Australia, into the contribution of chemotherapy to 5-year survival in 22 major adult malignancies, showed startling results: The overall contribution of curative and adjuvant cytotoxic chemotherapy to 5-year survival in adults was estimated to be 2.3% in Australia and 2.1% in the USA." [Royal North Shore Hospital Clin Oncol (R Coll Radiol) 2005 Jun;17(4):294.]

The research covered data from the *Cancer Registry* in Australia and the *Surveillance Epidemiology and End Results* in the USA for the year 1998. The current 5-year relative adult survival rate for cancer in Australia is over 60%, and no less than that in the USA. In comparison, a mere 2.3% contribution of chemotherapy to cancer survival does not justify the huge expense involved and the tremendous suffering patients experience because of severe, toxic side effects resulting from this treatment. With a meager success rate of 2.3%, selling chemotherapy as a medical treatment (instead of a scam), is one of the greatest fraudulent acts ever committed. The average chemotherapy earns the medical establishment a whopping $300,000 to $1,000,000 each year, and has so far earned those who promote this pseudo-medication (poison) over 1 trillion dollars. Medical doctors get $375,000 per patient for chemotherapy, radiation, x-ray, surgery, hospital stays, doctors and anesthesiologists, according statistics from the U.S. Department of Commerce. To earn such a large amount of money so easily can be very tempting to any doctor. However, a patient cured is a goldmine lost. It's no surprise that the medical establishment tries to keep this scam alive for as long as possible.

In 1990, the highly respected German epidemiologist, Dr. Ulrich Abel from the Tumor Clinic of the University of Heidelberg, conducted the most comprehensive investigation of every major clinical study on chemotherapy drugs ever done. Abel contacted 350 medical centers and asked them to send him anything they had ever published on chemotherapy. He also reviewed and analyzed thousands of scientific articles published in the most prestigious medical journals. It took Abel several years to collect and evaluate the data. Abel's epidemiological study, 'Chemotherapy of Advanced Epithelial Cancer: a critical review', Biomedicine and Pharmacotherapy, 1992; 46: 439-452., should have alerted every doctor and cancer patient about the risks of one of the most common treatments used for cancer and other diseases. In his paper, Abel came to the conclusion that the overall success rate of chemotherapy was "appalling." According to this report, **there was no scientific evidence available in any existing study to show that chemotherapy can "extend in any appreciable way the lives of patients suffering from the most common organic cancers."**

Abel points out that chemotherapy rarely improves the quality of life. He describes chemotherapy as "a scientific wasteland" and states that even though there is no scientific evidence that chemotherapy works, neither doctor nor patient is willing to give up on it. The mainstream media has never reported on this hugely important study, which is hardly surprising, given the enormous vested interests of the groups that sponsor the media, that is, the pharmaceutical companies. A recent search turned up exactly zero reviews of Abel's work in American journals, even though it was published in 1990. I believe this is not because his work was unimportant—but because it is irrefutable.

The truth of the matter would be far too costly for the pharmaceutical industry to bear, thus making it unacceptable. If the mass media reported the truth that medical drugs, including chemotherapy drugs, are used to practically commit genocide in the

U.S. and the world, their best sponsors (the pharmaceutical companies) would have to withdraw their misleading advertisements from the media – television, radio stations, magazines, and newspapers. But neither group wants to go bankrupt.

Many doctors go as far as prescribing chemotherapy drugs to patients for malignancies that are far too advanced for surgery, with the full knowledge that there are no benefits at all. Yet they claim chemotherapy to be an effective cancer treatment, and their unsuspecting patients believe that "effective" equals "cure." The doctors, of course, refer to the FDA's definition of an "effective" drug, one which achieves a 50% or more reduction in tumor size for 28 days. They neglect to tell their patients that there is no correlation whatsoever between shrinking tumors for 28 days and curing the cancer or extending life. **Temporary tumor shrinkage through chemotherapy has never been shown to cure cancer or to extend life.** In other words, you can live with an untreated tumor for just as long as you would with one that has been shrunken or eliminated by chemotherapy (or radiation). The bottom line is that tumors almost never kill anyone unless they obstruct the common bile duct or other vital passages. Certainly in primary cancer, the tumor is never health-endangering or life-threatening. And yet, it is treated as if it were the most dangerous thing on earth. All that progress made with regard to early tumor detection and successful shrinkage of tumors has not been able to increase the survival time of the cancer patient today to what is was 50 years ago. It is all too obvious that whatever standard medical treatment is used, it is the wrong treatment.

Besides, chemotherapy has never been shown to have curative effects for cancer. By contrast, the body can still cure itself, which it actually tries to do by developing cancer. Cancer is more a healing response than it is a disease. The "disease" **is** the body's attempt to cure itself of an existing imbalance. And sometimes, this healing response continues even if a person is subjected to chemotherapy (and/or radiation). Unfortunately, as the previously mentioned research has demonstrated, the chances for a real cure are greatly reduced when patients are treated with chemotherapy drugs.

The side effects of the treatment can be horrendous and heart-breaking for both patients and their loved ones, all in the name of trustworthy medical treatment. Although the drug treatment comes with the promise to improve the patient's quality of life, it is just common sense that a drug that makes them throw up and lose their hair, while wrecking their immune system, is doing the exact opposite. Chemotherapy can give the patient life-threatening mouth sores. It attacks the immune system by destroying billions of immune cells (white blood cells). Its deadly poisons inflame every part of the body. The drugs can slough off the entire lining of their intestines. The most common side effect experienced among chemo patients is their complete lack of energy. The new additional drugs now given to many chemo patients may prevent the patient from noticing some of the side effects, but they hardly reduce the immensely destructive and suppressive effect of the chemotherapy itself. Remember, the reason chemotherapy can shrink some tumors is because it causes massive destruction in the body.

If you have cancer, you may think that feeling tired is just part of the disease. This rarely is the case. Feeling unusually tired is more likely due to anemia, a common side effect of most chemotherapy drugs. Chemo drugs can dramatically decrease your red blood cell levels, and this reduces oxygen availability to the 60-100 trillion cells of your body. You can literally feel the energy being zapped from every cell of your body—a physical death without dying. Chemo-caused fatigue has a negative impact on day-to-day activities in 89% of all patients. With no energy, there can be no joy and no hope, and all bodily functions become subdued.

One long-term side effect is that these patients' bodies can no longer respond to nutritional or immune-strengthening approaches to cancerous tumors. All of this may explain why **cancer patients who do not receive any treatment at all, have an up to four times higher remission rate than those who receive treatment.** The sad thing is that chemotherapy does not cure 96% to 98% of all cancers anyway. Conclusive evidence (for the majority of cancers) that chemotherapy has any positive influence on survival or quality of life does not exist.

To promote chemotherapy as a treatment for cancer is misleading, to say the least. By permanently damaging the body's immune system and other important parts, chemotherapy has become a leading cause of treatment-caused diseases such as heart disease, liver disease, intestinal diseases, diseases of the immune system, infections, brain diseases, pain disorders, and rapid aging.

Before committing themselves to being poisoned, cancer patients need to question their doctors and ask them to produce the research or evidence that shrinking a tumor actually translates to any increase in survival. If they tell you that chemotherapy is your best chance of surviving, you will know they are lying or are simply misinformed. As Abel's research clearly demonstrated, there is no such evidence anywhere to be found in the medical literature. Subjecting patients to chemotherapy robs them of a fair chance of finding or responding to a real cure and deserves criminal prosecution.

What *Is* Cancer?

According to our current medical model, cancer is a general term that describes a group of 100 unique diseases that share one common factor: uncontrolled growth and spread of abnormal cells. Our body naturally produces more cells when it needs them. For example, every person who has done muscle training or exercised regularly knows that his muscles have become larger. However, we would not call the extra cell tissues that the body forms in response to an increased need for muscle power to be an abnormal growth or tumor. However, if cells begin to divide without an apparent need for more cells, they will form an excess mass of tissue which is considered a tumor. If the tumor is "malignant," doctors refer to it as cancerous.

For as long as the basic underlying mechanisms leading up to cancer are not known and dealt with properly, cancer will remain a mystery disease. Cancer is a puzzling phenomenon that has (falsely) been labeled an "autoimmune disease," a disease that allegedly turns the body against itself. The truth is far from that. The body has been designed to sustain its life for as long as possible. Even the so-called "death gene" has only one purpose, that is, to keep the body from self-destructing. Death genes are there to make sure cells die at the end of their normal lifespan and are replaced with new ones.

If the body is designed to live and not to destroy itself, why then would it suddenly allow the growth of extra cell tissue and kill itself? This does not make any sense at all. The main obstacle to finding real cures for cancer is that modern cancer treatment is rooted in the false assumption that the body sometimes tries to destroy itself. Medical students are trained to understand the mechanism of disease development, but they are left in the dark concerning the origins of disease. Viewed superficially, to the students, an illness appears to be something destructive and harmful to the body. Seen from a deeper perspective, however, the same illness is but an attempt by the body to cleanse and heal itself, or at least, to prolong its life. Since the medical textbooks offer few insights into the true causes of illness, it is understandable that the majority of doctors today believe that the body has self-destructive, and even suicidal abilities or tendencies. Claiming to be non-superstitious and objective, they inadvertently admit that certain cells suddenly decide to malfunction, become malicious, and randomly attack other cells and organs in the body. Based on this purely subjective and unsubstantiated belief, the doctor and his patient alike become almost obsessed with trying to protect the body from itself. Yet despite such undisputed notions of "truth," none of this means that the body does, in fact, attempt or cause its own destruction. Would it actually astound you if I told you that cancer has never killed a person?

Wisdom of Cancer Cells

Cancer cells are not part of a malicious disease process. When cancer cells "spread" (metastasize)[5] throughout the body, it is not

---

[5] It has never been proven that cancer cells move around the body and indiscriminately form new colonies of cancer cells. Rather, new colonies may grow for the same reasons the previous ones did.

their purpose or goal to disrupt the body's vitals functions, infect healthy cells, and obliterate their host (the body). Self-destruction is not the theme of any cell unless, of course, it is old, worn-out, and ready to be turned-over. Cancer cells, like all other cells, know that if the body dies, they will die as well. Just because most doctors and patients assume that cancer cells are out to destroy the body does not mean that cancer cells actually have such a purpose or ability. A cancerous tumor is neither the cause of progressive destruction nor does it actually lead to the death of the body. There is nothing in a cancer cell that even remotely has the ability to kill anything. If you asked people walking in the street if they knew how cancer kills people, you would probably not get one definite, correct answer. Ask the same question of doctors and you may not get a much better result. You will unlikely hear that cancer doesn't kill anyone.

Contrary to hearsay, what eventually leads to the demise of an organ or the entire body is the wasting away of healthy cell tissue, which results from a continued deprivation of nutrients and life force. **The drastic reduction or shutdown of vital nutrient supplies to the cells of an organ is not primarily a *consequence* of a cancerous tumor, but actually its biggest *cause*.**

By definition, a cancer cell is a normal, healthy cell that has undergone genetic mutation to the point that it can live in anaerobic surroundings (an environment where oxygen is not available). In other words, if you deprive a group of cells of vital oxygen (their primary source of energy), some of them will die, but others will manage to alter their genetic software program and mutate in a most ingenious way: the cells will become able to live without oxygen and will adapt to derive some of their energy needs from such things as cellular metabolic waste products (more about this in Chapter 2).

It may be easier to understand the cancer cells' phenomenon when comparing it with the behavior of common microorganisms. Bacteria, for example, are divided into two main groups, aerobic and anaerobic,[6] meaning, those that need to use oxygen

---

[6]There are some specialized bacteria that are both aerobic and anaerobic.

and those that can live without it. This is important to understand, since we have more bacteria in our body than we have cells. Aerobic bacteria thrive in an oxygenated environment. They are responsible for helping us with the digestion of food and with the manufacturing of important nutrients, such as B-vitamins. Anaerobic bacteria, on the other hand, can appear and thrive only in an environment where oxygen does not reach. They break down waste materials, toxic deposits, and dead, worn-out cells.

The Amazing Role of Germs and Infections

Destructive bacteria naturally increase in larger numbers wherever excessive waste matter accumulates and requires decomposition. Have you ever wondered why we have more bacteria in our body than we have cells? Most bacteria are produced inside the body, whereas relatively few enter it from the outside. The body also "grows" bacteria from tiny, indestructible colloids of life in our blood and cells. One of the world's most ingenuous medical researchers, Professor Antoine Bechamp (1816-1908), called these tiny cellular compounds *microzyma*. The German scientist, Dr. Günther Enderlein, who published papers on this research in 1921 and 1925, referred to them as *protits*. Protits are tiny dots in the blood and cells that you can apparently see with any microscope. These dots or colloids of life are virtually indestructible and survive even after the body dies.

According to the phenomenon known as *pleomorphism,* these protits develop or change form in response to a changing condition (acid/base balance) of the blood or cell milieu. As the cells' environment becomes acidified and toxic, the protits turn into microorganisms that are designed to break down and remove dead cells, toxins, and metabolic waste-products that the body is unable to remove. If further destruction of dead, weak cells and other waste is required, the protits become viruses and, eventually, fungi.

You may know how difficult it can be to get rid of a toe-nail/foot-fungus. Fungi only go after dead, organic matter. The presence of congested and half-decayed or dead toe tissue

34

practically forces the body to produce and/or attract more and more fungi to help decompose the lifeless parts of the foot.

As you might know, cancer cells are filled with all sorts of microorganisms. Allopathic medicine does not really explain how they get into the cells, unless they are viral. Most doctors assume that the germs come from the outside, but this assumption is unproved (and was even disputed by Louis Pasteur himself, who invented the germ theory).

As the brilliant scientists Bechamp and Enderlein demonstrated, these germs are created inside the cells in response to the presence of toxic waste material that the body is unable to remove. They may also attach themselves to other weak, undernourished cell tissue (particularly cells that suffer from poor oxygenation). Their purpose is to decompose these damaged, weak cells. This microbial activity is commonly known as "infection." Like cancer, however, an infection is not a disease. Rather, it is a sophisticated, combined attempt by the body and microbes to avert the suffocation and poisoning caused by accumulated toxic waste material in its tissues, the lymphatic system, or the blood.

If you piled up kitchen garbage in one area of your house, it would attract a lot of flies and bacteria, and this would generate a foul-smelling odor. You would certainly not blame the flies and bacteria for the stench. They are just trying to digest some of the garbage. Likewise, those microbes that are attracted to or produced inside unhealthy cells are not part of the problem; they are part of the solution to the problem.

An infection, if properly supported by natural approaches of cleansing and nourishment[7], can practically prevent the genetic mutation of aerobic cells into cancer cells. Cancer and infection share some of the same original causes. For this reason, a significant number of cancer patients who suffer a major infection such as the *chickenpox* go into total remission and are subsequently found cancer-free once the infection has passed. According to over 150 studies conducted in the past 100 or more years, spontaneous tumor regression has followed bacterial,

---

[7] See the author's book *Timeless Secrets of Health and Rejuvenation.*

fungal, viral, and protozoal infections.[8] During episodes of fever, tumors literally break up, and the cancer cells are promptly removed via the lymphatic system and other organs of elimination. During such a major infection—which is nothing but an appropriate healing response initiated by bacteria and the immune system—a considerable amount of toxic waste is broken down and removed from the body. This, once again, permits oxygen to reach the oxygen-deprived cells. Upon contact with the oxygen, the cancer cells die or otherwise mutate back into normal cells. The tumors have no more reason to be there, hence, the occurrence of spontaneous remission of cancer in these patients. In some cases, brain tumors as large as the size of an egg have literally disappeared in this way within 24 hours. The standard approach of suppressing infection and its resultant fever among hospital patients is medical malpractice and stands responsible for the loss of millions of lives that could easily have been saved by letting nature do its job.

Germs Don't Cause Cancer

The germs involved in an infection become active and infectious only when physical impurities and waste matter have gathered or tissue damage has already occurred. This is true whether they are of a bacterial or viral origin and whether they are generated within the body or introduced from the external environment. Destructive microorganisms (those involved in an infection) simply have no business in a clean, well-circulated, and oxygen-rich environment. There is nothing to be disposed of, and no immune response is necessary (fever, swelling of the lymph nodes, an increase of immune cells, or other such self-defensive measures) to protect the body.

Even if harmful germs were to enter cell tissue in a healthy

---

[8] Research paper by S. A. Hoption Cann, J. P. van Netten, and C. van Netten (July 2003)—Department of Healthcare and Epidemiology, University of British Columbia; Special Development Laboratory, Royal Jubilee Hospital and Department of Biology, University of Victoria, British Columbia, Canada.

body, they would do it no harm. A virus simply cannot penetrate into the nucleus of a well-oxygenated cell because exposure to oxygen would kill it. A well-oxygenated cell also produces powerful anti-viral drugs, such as *interferon*. If for some reason a virus has made contact with a cell, but its presence is not beneficial to the body, the virus will be destroyed by the cell's defense mechanisms or the general immune system. Viruses do not help cells mutate into cancer cells, unless this is in the best interest of the body. We should not fall into the trap of misinterpreting this to be an act of self-destruction. **It is important to recall at this point that cancer is not a disease but a survival mechanism that occurs only when all other protective measures have failed.**

There is profound purpose and intelligence at every level of physical creation, from the smallest of particles to the most complex star clusters in the large-scale universe. Just because many scientists and doctors prefer to see nature as behaving in a random, incoherent fashion does not mean it actually is chaotic and unpredictable. Cancer is not as chaotic as the "experts" would have us believe. It has as much purpose and meaning as does a virus or bacterium. A virus only infects the nucleus of a cell that is on the verge of becoming anaerobic. To find virus material in cancer cells is, therefore, not proof that viruses cause cancer. In fact, viruses try to prevent the demise of the body. They are created for the body and by the body. It is completely normal for weak, deteriorating cells to transform their protits colloids into bacteria, viruses, and fungi to help prevent more damage to the body than has already occurred due to the accumulation of toxic waste matter.

Suppressing an infection, such as chickenpox, with germ-killing medication destroys much of the germ population. However, it is the germ population that helps to stimulate a much-needed immune response to rid the body of cancer-causing toxins. Modern vaccination programs are largely responsible for the significant deterioration of natural immunity among the vaccinated populations around the world today. The body does not acquire real immunity to infectious diseases by exposing it to vaccines (antibody production alone does not create immunity);

in fact, with each vaccine the immune system becomes more depleted.

New vaccines that, for example, are said to prevent cervical cancer (connected with the human papillomavirus or HPV) merely force the body to move toxins into other areas. This may give rise to the appearance that the "enemy" is dead and the body is now cured and safe. Not by a long shot! The short-term gain of becoming symptom-free through the use of such magic bullet approaches can have serious repercussions in the long-term. These treatments aimed at producing a quick symptomatic relief actually prevent the body from employing the assistance of destructive microbes to help break down and remove deposits in the body that resemble nuclear waste.

The toxic waste and cell debris gathered in the body can act like a time bomb, but most people do not want to hear it ticking. They stick their heads in the sand, hoping that somehow the problem will simply go away. However, when the ticking becomes too unnerving and frightening (symptoms), the resulting visit to the doctor will lead to the smashing of the timing device, but will leave the bomb intact. Hence, it is just a matter of time before the bomb explodes; only this time, since the clock is now gone, there won't be much of a warning. On the other hand, allowing the body to receive assistance from destructive germs may not only defuse the time bomb but also dismantle it. The toxic secretions from these microbes prompt the immune system to launch a preemptive strike against potential cancer formation. A spontaneous remission of cancer is not a rare miracle. It happens in millions of people who unknowingly diffuse these "time bombs" through an infection, such as the simple cold or flu. This is how 95 percent of all cancers come and go without any medical intervention.

Based on current statistical information, we can estimate that treating cancer with suppressive methods, e.g. radiation, chemo-therapy, and surgery, reduces the chance of complete remission from 28% percent to 7% or less. In other words, medical treatment is responsible for the deaths of at least 21,000 people in every 100,000 cancer patients! These 21,000 people would recover if they did not receive any treatment at all. According to the American Cancer Society's estimated 2008 cancer mortality rates, 565,650 men and women will die from cancer this year (2008). That's 6,000 deaths more than in 2007. In a country that supposedly has the most advanced and successful medical system in the world, this trend clearly shows that the currently applied symptom-oriented approaches to cancer are heavily flawed and in fact, have failed.

Oh, These Bad Free Radicals!

Now imagine if we actually focused on removing the root causes of cancer. Wouldn't we find that cancer is actually not a threatening disease at all, and certainly not the killer disease we have been made to believe it is?

You may wonder about those bad *oxygen free radicals* that everyone talks about? Is it not true that they are behind most cancers and other diseases? If it is true, how can we defend ourselves against them, other than by removing them with such antioxidants as vitamin C?

Oxygen free radicals are highly reactive oxygen molecules. They are involved in causing rust in iron and in turning fats rancid. They are also found in arteries that have become occluded with plaque. Many researchers believe that free radicals are involved in the formation of cancer cells. However, like bacteria, free radicals have been given an unjustifiably bad reputation. Free radicals have existed since the beginning of life on Earth. Why would they now lead to cancer in one out of every two people when just 100 years ago only 1 in 8,000 people suffered the same fate? Did free radicals just become a lot more "vicious" in the past 100 years, ever so eager to oxidize us to death? The answer is a resounding "no."

Free radicals only oxidize and destroy what is already weak and potentially damaging to the body. They never attack healthy, vital cell tissue, but they naturally turn up where there is some-thing to be destroyed that has become useless and is an impending threat to the body's physiological balance. Weak or worn out cells and accumulated metabolic waste material, which the body's lymphatic system normally removes without a problem, become a hazard when they are trapped in the tissues and the free radicals are not doing their job. Increasing free radical activity and spreading infectious germs are therefore the next best alternatives to the body's own cleansing and eliminative efforts, especially when the body's immune system is already compromised. Thus, neither free radicals nor germs can rightfully be considered a **cause** of illness and aging. Since illness is actually a healing mechanism and aging is a form of advanced congestion in the body, free radicals must, in fact, be considered the beneficial **effects** of illness and aging.

The more often infections are "prevented" or suppressed through medical interventions, the less efficient the liver and kidneys, as well as the immune, lymphatic, and digestive systems become in keeping the body's cell tissues free of harmful, noxious deposits.

Yet, not only infections and free radicals act as cleansers or scavengers of obstructive waste and damaged, weak cells. Pain also serves as a healing aid. Pain is merely a signal that the body is actively involved in a healing response that includes repairing damaged tissues and cleansing itself. By suppressing pain with medication, you short-circuit the body's internal communication and healing mechanisms and practically force it to hold on to, and eventually suffocate in, its own waste. Cancer is a natural consequence of dealing with such a distressing, unnatural situation.

Mutated Genes Don't Cause Cancer

Cancer cells are normal, oxygen-dependent cells that have been genetically reprogrammed to survive in an oxygen-deprived environment. Why would a healthy cell nucleus, which contains the genetic makeup (DNA) of the cell, suddenly decide to give up its need for oxygen and turn itself into a cancer cell? This is a simple question that lies at the very the core of the complex mystery surrounding cancer. To resolve this mystery you have to change your idea about what cancer is. You are unlikely to find a satisfactory answer if you believe that cancer is an aggressive, life-threatening disease that spreads indiscriminately throughout the body, unless it is stopped or slowed by means of deadly drugs, radiation, or surgery. Those who know in their gut that the law of cause and effect applies to every natural phenomenon must wonder whether cancer is, after all, only the natural effect of an underlying, unnatural cause. To treat cancer as if it were an illness without removing its underlying cause is nothing but malpractice, that is, "bad or wrong practice." It is now clear that such an approach has potentially fatal consequences for most cancer patients. Instead of reducing cancer occurrence and cancer mortality, the current medical approaches used to treat cancer actually contribute to increasing both. Blaming the genes doesn't help.

The genetic blueprint in a cancerous cell is no longer aligned with the original genetic blueprint (DNA) found in other normal cells of the body. However, its genes didn't suddenly decide or volunteer to be "mal-aligned" or malignant, as they call it. Genetic blueprints do not act on anything, but when the cell environment changes, they become altered or mal-aligned with the original blueprints.

According to American research[9], the genes DNA-PK and p53 are essential components of the body's repair system. When they are intact, the cell is safe, but when either goes wrong, the cell divides and multiplies uncontrollably. DNA-PK normally repairs damaged genes. However, cancerous cells can also harness DNA-PK's power to repair themselves from damage caused by anti-cancer treatments. This makes these cells more resistant to the therapy, which may also explain why the orthodox cancer treatments, chemotherapy and radiotherapy, are such a failure. The more radical or intense the anti-cancer treatment is, the more "vicious" and powerful the cancer becomes; this, of course, dramatically reduces the chances for survival. It is similar to attacking a lion or water buffalo; the more aggressively you attack it, the more vicious the beast becomes. Likewise, repeatedly attacking bacteria with antibiotics makes them resistant to

---

[9] (*Cancer Research* 61, 8723-8729, December 15, 2001)

medical treatment. This results in the breeding of antibiotic-resistant organisms that are deadly and are acquired most often in places where antibiotics are administered frequently, and people's immune systems are the weakest, that is, in hospitals. This makes hospitals among the most dangerous places on earth.

Now, p53 acts as a signaling system, sending out messages that stop damaged cells from dividing and forming tumors. This powerful gene is altered in about 80 percent of cancers. However, the focus of cancer research should not be on figuring out what kind of genetic mutation occurs (genes showing up as faulty), but on the changes in the body that lead up to it. To repeat, genes do not just change without a reason. They only do so if they are forced to mutate in response to adverse changes in the cell environment.

Cancer—An Ingenious Rescue Mission

So what kind of extreme situation could possibly coerce a healthy cell to abandon its original genetic design and stop using oxygen? The answer is strikingly simple: a lack of oxygen. Normal cells meet their energy needs by combining oxygen with glucose. "Cell mutation" occurs only in surroundings where little or no oxygen is available. Without oxygen, the cells have to find other ways to meet their energy requirements.

The second most efficient option to obtain energy is through fermentation. Anaerobic cells (cancer cells) thrive in areas where plenty of metabolic waste products are trapped. These cells are capable of deriving energy from fermenting, for example, the metabolic waste product, lactic acid. This is similar to a starving animal eating its own excrement. By reusing lactic acid, the cancer cells accomplish two things. First, they derive energy for their sustenance and, second, they take this potentially dangerous waste product away from the immediate environment (the intercellular fluid or connective tissue) of the healthy cells. If cancer cells did not remove lactic acid from the cell environment, this extremely strong acid would accumulate and lead to fatal *acidosis*—a condition that involves the destruction of healthy cells due to high levels of acidity. Without the presence of a lactic acid-metabolizing tumor, the lactic acid could perforate the blood vessel walls and, along with other waste material and contaminants, enter the bloodstream. The result would be blood poisoning (septic shock) and subsequent death.

The body sees the cancer as such an important defense mechanism that it even causes the growth of new blood vessels to guarantee that the cancer cells receive a much-needed supply of glucose and, therefore, are able to survive and spread. It knows that the cancer cells do not cause, but prevent death, at least for a while, until the wasting away of an organ leads to the demise of the entire organism. If the trigger mechanisms for cancer (causal factors) are properly taken care of, such an outcome can be avoided.

Cancer is not a disease; it is the final and most desperate survival mechanism the body has at its disposal. It only takes control of the body when all other measures of self-preservation have failed. To truly heal cancer and what it represents in a person's life, we must come to the understanding that what the body does when allowing some of its cells to grow in abnormal ways is in its best interest. Cancer is not an indication that the body is about to destroy itself.

Chapter Two

Cancer's Physical Causes

Identifying the Origin of Cancer

To discover and understand the physical causes of cancer, you will first need to let go of the idea that cancer is a disease. You cannot have it both ways. Either you trust in your body's innate wisdom and healing abilities or you don't. In the former case you are already encouraged by what your body is doing on your behalf, and in the latter case you are frightened by it. The perspective of what cancer means to you ultimately determines whether you will heal or continue to fight an uphill battle.

The commonly held belief that cancer is a disease represents a powerful force that nearly every cancer patient is confronted with. Although this belief is based on a misconception of what cancer really is, it nevertheless generates a preoccupation with being healthy, which, in turn, further strengthens the belief of disease. Trying to be healthy shows that there exists an imbalance on all levels of body, mind and spirit. A balanced healthy person doesn't try to be healthy; he doesn't even think about it. Trying to be healthy requires a great deal of effort which is actually more an obstacle to being healthy than it is helpful. It prevents you from regaining your balance.

Healing is accepting, allowing, and supporting, not fighting or resisting. This is how spontaneous remissions occur. The body uses its maximum healing capacity when it is not preoccupied with a *fight or flight response* which occurs when you are under stress or feel threatened. As always, there is something to be learned from every situation, including having cancer. A person's willingness to face, accept and learn from the issues that cancer brings up turns this dis-ease into a purposeful, potentially uplifting, and sometimes even euphoric experience. During hundreds of interviews with cancer survivors over the past 30

44

years I found that almost all of them shared one experience: It had caused the most important and positive changes in their lives ever.

In our modern societies, we learn to go more by superficial appearances and less by the rather concealed larger picture of things. It is in the nature of life that for every symptom, an underlying cause exists, yet the cause lies hidden and seems to be unrelated to the symptom. Purely mechanistic approaches to treating the body, as they are applied in the system of allopathic medicine, usually fall short in locating and healing these hidden causes. They will remain undetected unless we begin to view the body as a *process* that is organized by a superb combination of energy and information or intelligence, rather than as an *assembly of different parts* such as we would find in a machine.

To treat the body as if it were composed merely of cells and molecules is akin to applying technology straight out of the Middle Ages to our present day world. Modern technologies and computers were derived from the principles of information and energy that came to light through the study of quantum physics; yet with regard to understanding the nature of life and treating the human body, we still rely mostly on old and outdated Newtonian principles. Understanding the way the human body operates becomes relatively easy once we apply the principles of quantum physics.

You as consciousness, soul or spirit, are the only true source of that energy and information that run your body. Your presence in the body and what you do, eat, drink, feel, and think determine how well your genes are able to control and sustain your physical existence. If you (the conscious presence) are no longer present in your body, the energy and information are withdrawn from every cell. We know this to be physical death. You are no longer present and your eyes are "empty." Seen from a superficial point of view, you could conclude that death has turned the body into a disordered heap of useless particles. Of course, if you had a wider perspective of death, you would be able to see it as the beginning of new life; all the atoms that previously comprised these cells have simply relocated themselves to assemble once again in new forms, such as air, water, soil, plants, fruit, animals or other human beings. Therefore, life does not end with death; only the form changes. Besides, your consciousness remains unaffected by all of this because it is not physical (even if living in a physical body) and cannot be destroyed.

Now, if you only partially withdrew your energy and purposeful connectedness from some parts of your body, would those parts not move into disarray and chaotic behavior? This is what medicine calls disease, meaning, you are no longer in ease or alignment with the orderly fashion in which the body normally operates. However, as you will begin to realize, disease is only an illusion of perception. Like death, disease is nothing but the provider of new life. **Yet unlike death, disease offers us the opportunity to restore our life while remaining in this physical form.** Cancer only strikes when a part or parts of us are not alive anymore, physically, emotionally, and spiritually. Cancer can resurrect these numbed, suppressed, or congested areas, whether they are physical or non-physical in nature.

The resurrection, which begins with increased attention to these dead zones of our life, can occur in a number of ways. We may gradually become aware how afraid or negligent we are of a particular body part, the body as a whole, our future or our past, nature, food, other people, the future of our planet, or other issues. Suddenly, we may begin to realize how deeply we have harbored intense negative emotions toward others or ourselves, or we may notice why we have allowed certain foods, beverages, or drugs such as painkillers, steroids, and antibiotics to contaminate and congest our beautiful body. Cancer is a wakeup call, prompting us to take our life back when it no longer feels meaningful. The alarm bell that sounds to wake us up rings painfully loud, which is good because we are more likely to respond to physical than to emotional pain.

The "disease" cancer occurs only where channels or ducts of circulation and elimination have been consistently blocked for a long time. This chapter deals with the purely physical causes of cancer, although, to truly make sense of cancer, it must also be seen in the context of emotional and spiritual causes. These are the subject matter of Chapters Three and Four.

Cancer's Progressive Stages

Since I am writing this book mainly for the layperson, I will omit the typical medical jargon and references to complicated-sounding scientific studies that so obscure the subject matter of cancer. Instead, I will explain in simple step-by-step terms how most cancers develop. You will see the common thread that connects the symptom, cancer, with its layers of origin. Together we will unravel the mystery of cancer by going through its progressive stages in reverse order. Please keep in mind that each cause is just another effect of yet another cause. Eventually, though, we will arrive at the root origin of cancer, which I will explain in Chapter Four.

I have mentioned before that a cancer cell is one that has lost the ability to fulfill its preprogrammed responsibilities of ensuring balance or homeostasis in the body. Instead of fulfilling its natural duty, such a cell has turned itself over to a new line of professional occupation that you could describe as "sewer worker." It is not a coincidence or bad luck, but a necessity and a blessing in disguise, that cancer cells grab hold of and ingest harmful byproducts of metabolism. As we shall see, this waste material has no means to escape the cell surroundings, except via the "hungry mouths" of cancer cells.

A common consensus among the majority of the medical and lay population holds that the gradual "degradation" of normal cells into cancer cells is due to random mistakes that the body somehow makes, perhaps because of hereditary reasons, often called genetic predisposition. This theory not only defies logic, but also the intrinsic purpose of evolution.

Every great discovery man has made has revealed that something seemingly useless or even harmful is actually imbued with meaning and purpose. The destruction of the blossoms of a fruit tree should not to be mistaken as an act of self-annihilation; rather it is the destructive force that brings nutritious fruit to life. Although the idea that cancer is a deadly weapon the body creates to destroy itself (an autoimmune disease) is based on medical tests, it does not reflect a high degree of scientific insight and certainly defies all sense of wisdom and logic. Do we need a new, different interpretation of these tests to actually make sense of cancer and why it occurs?

As mentioned earlier, in 1900 only one in 8,000 people had cancer. Now one in every two people can expect to develop some type of cancer during his or her lifetime. In the United States alone, nearly one million people die each year from a chronic illness, most of them from cancer. Cancer has recently surpassed heart disease as the number one cause of death. What is going on here? Nothing in the natural world and its history suggests that such a mass exodus is normal. An old proverb says, "A little knowledge is a dangerous thing." Nowhere is this more true than with regard to our present knowledge of cancer. If we wish to halt and reverse the current cancer epidemic, we need to expand our horizon of knowledge. Not knowing what cancer really is has made it into a dangerous disease.

During every single day in your adult life, the body turns over about 30 billion cells. Out of these, an estimated one percent become damaged in the process and turn cancerous. Your immune system is programmed to detect these cells and destroy them through a highly sophisticated arsenal of weapons, including T-killer cells. The body's "clean-up task force" is so efficient, perfectly timed, and thorough that cancer cells stand no chance of surviving. Yet, it is essential for the body's own survival that these kinds of cancer cells are created everyday; they make certain that the immune system remains stimulated enough to keep its defense and self-purification capability efficient and up-to-date.

This naturally raises the question of why the same immune system would refrain from attacking cancer cells that have mutated in response to dealing with severe congestion (as explained below). Let me ask the same question in a different way. Why does the immune system discriminate between these two kinds of cancers and decide to destroy one group of cancer cells while leaving the other unharmed?

This important question deserves an answer. The cancer we generally refer to as disease is not actually a disease at all; rather it is an extended immune response to help clear up an existing

48

condition of congestion that suffocates a group of cells. Why would the immune system try to hinder the body's own efforts to prevent certain toxic metabolic waste products from entering the bloodstream and killing the body? Given the circumstances, these cancer cells are far too precious and too useful for the body to eliminate them. Even if they entered the lymphatic ducts and were transported to other parts of the body,[10] the immune system would still try to keep them alive for as long as they were useful. Cancer cells do not randomly spread throughout the body. They lodge themselves in places that are also congested, places that are oxygen-deprived.

Both healthy and cancerous cells in the body are loaded with cancer-killing white cells, such as T-cells. In the case of kidney cancer and melanomas, for example, white cells make up 50 per cent of the mass of the cancers. Since T-cells easily recognize foreign or mutated cell tissue such as cancer cells, you would expect these immune cells to attack cancer cells right away. However, the immune system allows cancer cells to recruit it to actually grow larger tumors and develop tumors in others parts of the body as well. Cancer cells produce specific proteins that tell the immune cells to leave them alone and help them to grow.

Why would the immune system want to collaborate with cancer cells to make more or larger tumors? Because cancer is a survival mechanism, not a disease. The body uses the cancer to keep deadly carcinogenic substances and caustic metabolic waste matter away from the lymph and blood and, therefore, from the heart, brain, and other vital organs. Killing off cancer cells would in fact jeopardize its survival.

It is important to know that the body attacks a cancerous tumor only after the congestion that has led to the tumor's growth in the first place has been broken up. As mentioned in Chapter One, this would be the case, for example, following a major infection, such as the chickenpox or the flu. I will discuss other reasons for the occurrence of spontaneous remissions at a later

---

[10] This is called metastasis. However, there is no evidence to show that metastasis really occurs. It is more likely that a "new" cancer develops in other parts of the body for the same reasons the first cancer developed.

stage in this book.

1. Congestion

The most pressing question is what kind of congestion are we talking about here and where is it coming from? Allow me to illustrate by using the following example: In a big city like New York, traffic may flow smoothly during normal hours or on Sundays, but at rush hour there are suddenly far more cars on the road than the city can handle. The resulting traffic congestion may force you to spend hours instead of minutes getting from your work place to your home. Eventually, though, you will find your way home. This is what I call temporary congestion. However, the situation would be different if there had been a major traffic accident due to ice and snow, and the roads leading to your home were now completely blocked. This accident affects every car waiting to move forward, although nothing is inherently wrong with the cars themselves. Equally affected are trucks that deliver goods to stores or take trash to landfills; mothers on their way home to feed their children; businessmen heading to the airport to catch a plane; and thousands of other commuters stranded for various reasons. The effect is the same for all involved; they are unable to reach their destination. Unless someone removes the cause of the traffic congestion, they remain stuck among a vast number of exhaust-producing cars.

If someone were to come along and propose that the best way to clear the congestion would be to get a large bulldozer and push every car off the road, you would think he must be out of his mind. Yet, this is exactly how allopathic medicine deals with cancer. In cancer, a more or less a permanent traffic jam has developed in the body, but this traffic jam has been caused by a holdup somewhere else. No longer can nutrients, such as oxygen and glucose, be delivered to their destinations, nor can cellular waste products be cleared away. Instead of using toxic drugs or surgical "bulldozers" to destroy or remove cells that have been affected by the traffic congestion, seeking the initial holdup that has led to the congestion in the first place would be a far wiser course of action.

We have already analyzed that normal cells turn cancerous when they do not get enough oxygen to do their metabolic work. Without cell metabolism, the body would turn cold and lifeless within minutes.

To keep some sort of metabolism going without the use of oxygen, albeit far from ideal, the cells have to change (mutate) into anaerobic cells that are capable of utilizing accumulated metabolic waste products and delivering at least some of the required heat and energy in the body. To blame and, subsequently, punish these cells for such an act of instinctive wisdom would be very shortsighted. If you look for the underlying reason for this situation, it is the holdup that prevents oxygen and other nutrients from reaching the cells. There is basically only one such holdup, although it has two components—the thickening of the blood capillary walls and the congestion of the lymphatic ducts.

2. The Holdup

Please be reminded that we are trying to trace the origin(s) of cancer, step by step, moving from the symptom toward the cause. The holdup that causes a traffic jam is apparently due to the wreck of a car or truck, but in reality, it is brought about by another factor, such as fatigue, distraction due to talking on a cell phone, speeding, or drunken driving. In the human body, such a holdup can be generated by thickened blood vessel walls, which prevent the proper passage of oxygen, water, glucose, and other vital nutrients from the blood to the cells.

Nutrients in the blood naturally pass through the blood vessel wall and gravitate to the cells through a process known as *osmosis*. After dropping off its precious cargo, the blood returns to the lungs, liver, and digestive system to take up more of the same. Some nutrients, such as water and oxygen, pass through the blood vessel walls freely, whereas others need assistance in the form of a carrier or guide. The hormone insulin, secreted by specialized pancreatic cells, plays such a role. It is released when any of several stimuli are detected. These include protein ingestion, and presence of glucose in the blood. Once injected into the blood by the pancreas, insulin takes up sugar (in the form of glucose) from the blood and transports it into muscle, fat, and liver cells, where it is converted into energy (ATP) or stored as fat. This basic metabolic process, which is responsible for keeping the entire body alive and healthy, becomes disturbed once the blood vessel walls begin to thicken.

Why would the body allow its blood vessel walls to become thicker? The answer may shock you: to save it from suffering a heart attack, stroke, or other form of sudden degeneration.

The most important fluid in the body is the blood. Its high velocity and thinness guarantee the continued sustenance of the body. If the blood gets too thick, the entire body, including the heart and the brain, begin to suffer oxygen deprivation and potential starvation. In thickened blood, platelets become aggravated and begin to stick together. This makes it difficult for the blood to pass through the tiny capillaries that supply the cells of the body with oxygen and other nutrients. If brain cells, nerve tissue, or heart cells get cut off from the oxygen and nutrient supply, a whole range of acute and chronic disorders may result, including heart attack, stroke, multiple sclerosis, fibromyalgia, Alzheimer's disease, Parkinson's disease, cancer of the brain, and many subsidiary problems throughout the body.

Given the vital importance of the blood, the body tries to ensure that the blood stays thin under all circumstances. In fact, the body employs numerous blood-thinning techniques and systems to prevent the dangerous thickening of its life-giving juice. I will, however, focus on only one of them because it is directly related to the thickening of blood vessel walls, and it is hardly ever recognized as a cause of cancer and many other degenerative disorders.

The Protein-Cancer Connection

The protein-cancer connection has become obvious ever since large-scale scientific studies, including the "China Study," have demonstrated a virtual absence of cancer among people who don't eat animal proteins. Meat consumption in relation to cancer risk has been reported in over a hundred epidemiological studies from many countries with diverse diets. Based on Richard Doll and Richard Peto's work in 1981 (*J Natl Cancer Inst.* 1981;66:1191–1308.), it has been estimated that approximately 35% (range 10%–70%) of cancer can be attributed to diet, similar in magnitude to the contribution of smoking to cancer (30%, range 25%–40%). Recently, a large American study has provided strong evidence that the consumption of red and processed meats poses the greatest dietary risk of developing cancer.

In a National Institutes of Health (NIH)-AARP Diet and Health Study, researchers Genkinger and Koushik from the U.S. National Cancer Institute examined the health data of 494,000 participants. In this 8-year study (published in *PLoS Med.* 2007 December; 4(12): e345, and online 2007 Dec. 11. doi:10.1371/journal.pmed.0040345), the researchers compared the rate of cancer occurrence among the 20 percent of participants who ate the most red and processed meat[11] with the data on the 20 percent who ate the least.

The results of the study were dramatic. Participants who consumed the most red meat had a 25 percent higher risk of developing colorectal cancer compared with those who ate the least, and a 20 percent higher risk of developing lung cancer.[12] The risk of esophageal and liver cancer was increased by between 20 and 60 percent. Higher meat intake also correlated with an increased risk or pancreatic cancer in men. In recent meta-analyses of colorectal cancer that included studies published up to 2005, summary associations indicated that red meat intakes were associated with 28%–35% increased risks while processed meats were associated with elevated risks of 20%–49%.

The researchers indicated that 1 in 10 cases of lung or colorectal cancer could be averted by limiting red meat intake. According to the China study and other cancer research consid-

---

[11]Meat originating from a mammal, beef, lamb, pork, and veal; and meats preserved by salting, smoking, or curing.
[12] Lung and colorectal cancers are the first and second leading causes of cancer death, respectively.

ered during the past 60 years, cancer could actually become a rare illness if animal proteins were avoided altogether.

Other studies have found associations between meat intake and the risk of bladder, breast, cervical, endometrial, esophageal, glioma, kidney, liver, lung, mouth, ovarian, pancreatic and prostate cancers. On the other hand, there are plenty of studies that point to the cancer-preventing effects of a fruit and vegetable diet, including recent studies published in the *American Journal of Epidemiology* 2007 Jul 15;166(2):170-80. Epub 2007 May 7 and Archives of Internal Medicine 2007 Dec 10;167(22):2461-8.

The researchers of the NIH diet study suggested that meat contains a number of carcinogenic compounds, including some that are formed during cooking or processing (e.g. heterocyclic amines, nitrosamines). They also noted that meat contains other potential carcinogens, including heme iron (the type of iron found in meat), nitrates and nitrites, saturated fat, antibiotics, hormones, and salts. All of these substances have been observed to affect hormone metabolism, increase cell proliferation, damage DNA, encourage insulin-like growth hormones and promote damage of cells by free radicals, all of which can lead to cancer. Children who eat processed meats increase their risk of developing leukemia by 74 percent, according to research published in the journal *BMC Cancer* (Jan. 2009).

What actually happens when you eat meat?

The most blood-thickening agent is food protein, particularly if it is derived from an animal source. Let us assume you eat a medium-sized piece of steak, chicken or fish (cadaver protein). When compared to a carnivorous animal like a lion or a wolf, your stomach can produce only the relative amount of 1/20 of the hydrochloric acid needed to digest such a concentrated protein meal. In addition, the relative concentration of the hydrochloric acid in cats or wolves is at least five times higher than in humans. A cat or wolf can easily eat and digest the bones of a chicken, whereas humans cannot. Most of the cadaver's protein, therefore, will pass undigested into the small intestine where it will either putrefy (80%) or enter the bloodstream (20%).

The liver is able to break down some of the absorbed protein, which forms the waste products urea and uric acid. This waste matter is passed on to the kidneys for excretion with the urine. However, with regular consumption of animal proteins, including meat, poultry, fish, eggs, cheese, and milk, more and more intrahepatic stones are formed in the bile ducts of the liver.[13] This greatly reduces the liver's ability to break down these proteins.

Protein foods are among the most acid-forming and blood-thickening foods of all. Therefore, when a major portion of the protein ends up circulating in the blood, it will, of course, thicken the blood. To avoid the danger of a heart attack or stroke, the body will attempt to dump the protein into the fluid surrounding the cells (tissue fluid or connective tissue). This thins the blood and averts the imminent danger of serious cardiovascular complications, at least for the time being. However, the dumped protein begins to turn the intercellular fluid into a gel-like substance. In this condition, nutrients that are trying to make their way to the cells may be caught in the thick soup, which increases the risk of cell death due to starvation.

The body tries to avoid cell death by initiating another, even more sophisticated, survival response, which is next to ingenious. To remove the proteins from the intercellular fluid, the body rebuilds the protein and converts it into collagen fiber, which is 100% protein. (See Illustration 1.) In this form, the body is able to build the protein into the basal membrane of the blood vessel walls. While accommodating the excessive protein, the basal membrane may become up to eight times as thick as is normal. Once, the capillary walls are saturated with the protein or collagen fiber, the basal membranes of the arteries start doing the same. This eventually, leads to a hardening of the arteries, which is the subject matter of Chapter Nine of my book, *Timeless Secrets of Health and Rejuvenation.*[14]

---

[13] See *The Amazing Liver and Gallbladder Flush* for details on the causes of stones in the bile ducts and gallbladder and how to remove them safely and painlessly.

[14] This book discusses in depth the causes of heart disease, strokes, and high cholesterol, and shows the reader how to remove these causes quickly and safely.

Now the body must face an even greater challenge. The thick walls of the capillaries (and possibly, the arteries) have become an obstruction, blocking the nutrient supply to the cells. The blood vessel walls increasingly prevent oxygen, glucose, and even water from penetrating the protein barricades, thus depriving cells of their bare nutrient essentials. Less glucose makes its way to the cells. As a result, cell metabolism drops to a lower level of efficiency, and waste production increases, similar to a car engine that has not been tuned properly or given quality gas or oil.

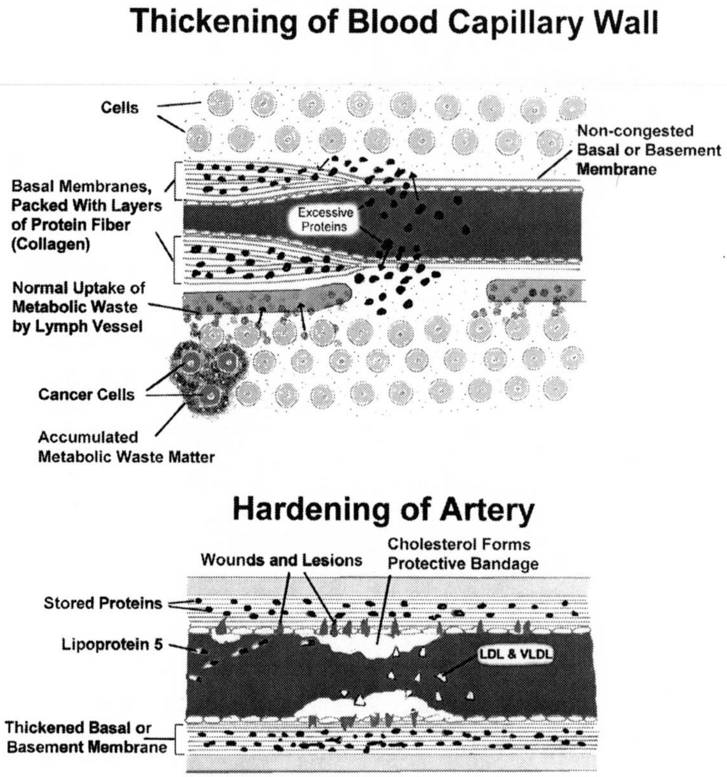

Thickening of Blood Capillary Wall

Hardening of Artery

Illustration 1: Cancer and Heart Disease Share the Same Cause

In addition to congesting the blood vessel walls, another complicating factor comes into play. Part of the excessive protein is absorbed by the lymphatic ducts that accompany every blood capillary. These lymph ducts and their attached lymph nodes are designed to remove and detoxify the normal amounts of cell-generated metabolic waste products. They also take away the cellular debris resulting from the daily destruction of over 30 billion worn-out cells. Since cells are composed of proteins, much of the collected waste is already filled with old cell protein. Being forced to take up extra protein from ingested foods like meat, fish, or milk simply overtaxes the entire lymphatic system and leads to the stagnation of lymph flow and fluid retention. Consequently, the congested lymph ducts are increasingly disabled as they attempt to take up the cells' metabolic waste products. This, in turn, leads to a higher concentration of metabolic waste material in the fluid surrounding the cells.

Suffocation in Progress

The consequence of waste buildup in the cell environment is that cells not only become deprived of oxygen and other vital nutrients, but they also begin to suffocate in their own waste. The dramatic change of the cell environment leaves them with no other choice but to mutate into "abnormal" cells, given the circumstances.

Cell mutation does not occur because the genes of the cell had a bad day and decided to play malignant. Genes do not switch themselves on and off without a reason. Genetic blueprints have no control or power to do anything. They are merely there to help the cell reproduce itself. However, the genetic blueprint becomes naturally altered when the environment of the cell undergoes major changes. By drastically reducing the concentration of oxygen in the cell environment, out of necessity the genes generate a new blueprint that enables them to survive without oxygen and instead use some of the metabolic waste products for energy. Mutated cells can take up, for example, lactic acid, and by metabolizing it, they are able to cover some of their energy needs. Although this abnormal type of cell metabolism has harmful side effects, by doing this, the body can avert, at least for a little while, the fatal poisoning of the affected organ or the blood. By keeping at least some of the oxygen-deprived cells alive through cell mutation, the organ is safeguarded against irreversible and sudden collapse and failure. **All of these adaptations make cancer a survival mechanism to keep the person alive for as long as circumstances permit.**

Cancer and Heart Disease—Same Causes

It is worth mentioning at this point that only capillary and arterial walls can store excessive protein. Venules and veins, unlike capillaries and arteries, are responsible for taking up the metabolic waste product carbon dioxide and carrying it toward the lungs. They basically carry "empty handed" blood, blood that has already *off-loaded* its nutrients and excessive protein and passed these into the connective tissues (the fluid surrounding the cells). The blood is now ready to return to the lungs to take up oxygen, carbon, nitrogen, and hydrogen molecules from the air. These four molecules make up all the amino acids in the body that are required for the building of cell proteins.[15] As the blood passes through the digestive system, it takes up other nutrients needed for energy and cell nourishment, and perhaps proteins from an animal source.

Concentrated proteins as found, for example, in meat, fish, poultry, eggs, cheese and milk are never stored in the walls of venules and veins, only in the walls of capillaries and arteries. Protein deposits in the basal membranes[16] of the capillaries and arteries injure and inflame the cells that make up these blood vessels. To deal with these injuries or lesions, the body attaches protective plaque, including cholesterol, to the interior of the artery wall in order to prevent dangerous blood clots from escaping into the bloodstream and triggering a heart attack or stroke. Venules and veins, on the other hand, always remain free

---

[15] More details about the protein self-sufficiency of the body in the section on vegetarianism of *Timeless Secrets of Health and Rejuvenation*.

[16] A normally very thin membrane that supports the cells comprising the blood vessel wall and keeps them in place.

of plaque because their basal membranes are not exposed to the damaging proteins. For this reason, heart surgeons are able to take veins from the legs, and use these as bypasses for arterial blockages. However, once put in the place of a coronary artery, a vein becomes just as exposed to excessive protein, and as a result, begins to develop protective plaque along its interior wall.

Cholesterol-containing plaque has gotten a bad name because not many physicians are aware of its real purpose. If more people knew that "bad" cholesterol (LDL) prevents bleeding of congested artery walls and, possibly, life-endangering blood clot formation, we might perceive "bad" cholesterol as life-saving cholesterol. By asking your doctor why the "bad" cholesterol attaches itself only to arteries and not to veins, although it is present in both venous and arterial blood, you may stir some curiosity in him as to why cholesterol acts in this manner. He may discover that cholesterol is not the enemy here. In fact, the body uses LDL cholesterol in the healing of every wound, internal and external. LDL cholesterol is truly a life saver.

I bring up the topic of hardening of the arteries because heart disease and cancer are not such radically different forms of illness or, to say it more accurately, survival mechanisms. They share two common factors: blood vessel wall congestion and lymphatic blockage. Since heart cells cannot become cancerous, once they are deprived of oxygen for a certain period of time, they die of acidosis and simply shut down. We refer to this as a heart attack, although in reality there is no attack, just oxygen deprivation. In other parts of the body a similar oxygen-deprived environment will result in some cells that are able to continue living, but not without undergoing mutation into cancer cells. In other words, cancer of the tissues can only occur in the body if the circulatory system (including both the blood and lymph vessels) has suffered from congestion for a long time.

Death in Trans Fats

Protein is not the only reason that cancer-causing congestion occurs. Certain fats known as trans fatty acids, or trans fats, attach themselves to the cell membranes, thereby making it difficult for the cells to receive enough oxygen, glucose, and even water. Oxygen-deprived, dehydrated cells become damaged and turn cancerous.

In particular, one's consumption of polyunsaturated fats as contained in refined and vitamin E depleted products, such as thin vegetable oil, mayonnaise, salad dressings, and most brands of margarine, leads to a particularly high risk for the development of skin cancer and most other cancers. Since most animal protein foods also contain fats that are exposed to high heat during food preparation, or even contain added fats as, for example, in fried chicken or fish sticks, the risk of cancer rises dramatically when these food items are combined and eaten regularly. The bottom line is that concentrated protein foods and refined fats hinder oxygen from entering the cells.

According to *Archives of Internal Medicine*, 1998, eating polyunsaturated fats increases the risk of breast cancer by 69 percent. By contrast, ingesting monounsaturated fats, as found in olive oil, reduces breast cancer risk by 45 percent.

This phenomenon is easy to understand. Once in contact with air, polyunsaturated fats attract many oxygen free radicals and become oxidized, that is, they turn rancid. Oxygen free radicals are generated when oxygen molecules lose an electron. This makes them highly reactive. Eating these aggressive fats causes them to attach to cell membranes in a manner similar to an oil slick in the sea engulfing and suffocating birds and sea creatures. Thus, the free radical activity in such fats has a severely damaging effect on cells, tissues, and organs.

Oxygen free radicals can form in refined, polyunsaturated oils and fats once they are exposed to air and sunlight before consumption. The free radicals may also form in the tissues after the oils or fats have been ingested. Polyunsaturated fats are difficult to digest, since they are deprived of their natural bulk and are no longer protected against free radicals by their natural protector, vitamin E, a powerful antioxidant; this important vitamin is being removed during the refining process. Eating a hamburger and French fries, for example, can flood your body with free radicals. However, blaming free radicals for causing damage in the body is like blaming the bullets for a shooting victim's injuries when, in fact, the person who pulled the trigger is responsible.

Saturated fats are solid and found in products such as lard and butter. They contain large quantities of natural antioxidants, which make them much safer against oxidation by free radicals. Since polyunsaturated fats are manufactured and do not exist in natural form, they are indigestible, and the body recognizes them as dangerous. Margarine, for example, is just one molecule away from plastic, and therefore extremely difficult to digest. Free radicals, which are the body's natural cleansers, try to get rid of the fatty culprits that have affixed themselves to the cell membranes. When the radicals digest these harmful fats, they also damage the cell membranes. This is considered to be a main cause of aging and degenerative disease.

Research has shown that out of 100 people who consumed large quantities of polyunsaturated fats, 78 showed marked clinical signs of premature aging. They also looked much older than others of the same age did. By contrast, in a recent study on the relationship between dietary fats and the risk for developing Alzheimer's disease, researchers were surprised to learn that the natural, healthy fats can actually reduce the risk for Alzheimer's by up to 80 percent. The study showed that the group with the lowest rate of Alzheimer's ate approximately 38 grams of these healthy fats every day, while those with the highest incidence of this disorder consumed only about half of that amount.

Cells that are damaged by abnormal free radical activity are unable to reproduce properly and this can impair major functions in the body, including those of the immune, digestive, nervous, and endocrine systems. Ever since polyunsaturated fats were introduced to the population on a large scale, degenerative diseases have increased dramatically, skin cancer being one of them. In fact, polyunsaturated fats have even made sunlight "dangerous," something that never would have been the case if foods hadn't been altered and manipulated by the food industry as they are today.[17] When polyunsaturated fats are removed from

---

[17] See more details in Andreas Moritz's book, *Heal Yourself with Sunlight* or *Timeless Secrets of Health and Rejuvenation*.

their natural foods, they need to be refined, deodorized, and even hydrogenated, depending on the food product for which they are used. During this process some of the polyunsaturated fats undergo chemical transformations, which turn them into *trans fatty acids* (trans fats), often referred to as "hydrogenated vegetable oils." Margarine may be composed of up to 54 percent trans fatty acids while a typical vegetable shortening can be 58 percent trans fats.

You can detect hydrogenated vegetable oils in foods by reading the labels. Most processed foods contain them, including breads, crisps, chips, doughnuts, crackers, biscuits, pastries, almost all baked goods, cake and frosting mixes, baking mixes, frozen dinners, sauces, frozen vegetables, and breakfast cereals. In other words, nearly all foods that are shelved, processed, refined, preserved, and not fresh can contain trans fats. They inhibit the cell's ability to use oxygen, which is required to burn foodstuffs to carbon dioxide and water. Of course, cells that are inhibited in completing their metabolic processes are likely to become cancerous.

Trans fats also make the blood thicker by increasing the stickiness of platelets. This multiplies the chances of blood clots and the build-up of fatty deposits, which can lead to heart disease. Researchers at Harvard Medical School, who observed 85,000 women over eight years, found that those eating margarine had an increased risk of coronary heart disease. A Welsh study linked the concentration of these artificial trans fats in body fat with death from heart disease. The Dutch government has already banned any products containing trans fatty acids.

Why is an increased risk of heart disease so important in the consideration of cancer? It is because cancer and heart disease share the same causes. A heart attack occurs when a part of the heart muscle is deprived of oxygen and dies. Cancer occurs when a part of an organ or system in the body is deprived of oxygen and would die if the body's cells were not able to mutate and become cancerous. If the blockages leading up to oxygen starvation are not removed, either cancer or heart failure is most likely going to take the person's life. Oftentimes, cancer patients do not actually die because of the cancer, but due to a failing heart. In my experience with hundreds of cancer patients, I found that all of them also suffered from major cardiovascular problems.

It is not a new discovery that chronic oxygen deprivation of cells is behind cancer and other degenerative disorders such as heart disease. During the 1930s, Otto Warburg, M.D., discovered that cancer cells have a lower-than-normal respiration rate compared to normal cells. He reasoned that cancer cells thrived in a low-oxygen environment and that increased oxygen levels would harm and even kill them. Winner of the 1931 Nobel Prize in Medicine, Dr. Warburg summarized the cancer problem in two short sentences: "Cancer has only one prime cause. It is the replacement of normal oxygen respiration of the body's cells by an anaerobic cell respiration."

Other scientists soon followed in Warburg's footsteps.

"Lack of oxygen clearly plays a major role in causing cells to become cancerous." - *Dr. Harry Goldblatt, Journal of Experimental Medicine, 1953*

"Insufficient oxygen means insufficient biological energy that can result in anything from mild fatigue to life threatening disease. The link between insufficient oxygen and disease has now been firmly established." - *Dr. W. Spencer Way, Journal of the American Association of Physicians (Dec. 1951)*

"Oxygen plays a pivotal role in the proper functioning of the immune system; i.e. resistance to disease, bacteria and viruses." - *Dr. Parris Kidd*

"In all serious disease states we find a concomitant low oxygen state . . . Low oxygen in the body tissues is a sure indicator for disease . . . Hypoxia, or lack of oxygen in the tissues, is the fundamental cause for all degenerative disease." - *Dr. Stephen Levine, Renowned Molecular Biologist*

"Cancer is a condition within the body where the oxidation has become so depleted that the body cells have degenerated beyond physiological control." - *Dr. Wendell Hendricks, Hendricks Research Foundation*

"Starved of oxygen the body will become ill, and if this persists it will die. "I doubt if there is any argument about that." - *Dr. John Muntz, Nutritional Scientist*

"He who breathes most air lives most life" - *Elizabeth Barrett Browning*

3. Lymphatic Blockage

What is lymph and why is it so vitally important in the body? Lymph originates as blood plasma, which is packed with all sorts of "groceries," including oxygen, glucose, minerals, vitamins, hormones, proteins, as well as antibodies and white blood cells. Blood plasma passes through the blood capillary walls and joins the tissue fluid that surrounds all the cells. Tissue fluid is also known as *intracellular fluid, interstitial fluid* or *connective tissue.* The cells take up nutrients from, and release metabolic waste products into, the tissue fluid. About 90 percent of the tissue fluid returns to the blood stream where it again becomes blood plasma. The remaining 10 percent of the tissue fluid forms what is called *lymph.* With the exception of carbon dioxide, lymph contains all the metabolic waste produced by the cells, as well as pathogens, dissolved proteins, and cancer cells (which are naturally generated as part of the normal turnover of cells). Lymph capillaries take up the lymph and remove this "trash," thereby preventing suffocation and damage of cells.

The degree of nourishment, health and efficiency of the cells depends on how swiftly and completely waste material is removed from the tissue fluid, now lymph. Since most cellular waste products cannot pass directly into the blood for excretion, they must gather in the tissue fluid until they are removed by the lymphatic system. Lymph vessels carry this potentially harmful material into the lymph nodes for filtration and detoxification.

Lymph nodes, which are strategically located throughout the body, also remove some fluid. This prevents the body from swelling and gaining excessive weight.

One of the key functions of the lymphatic system is to keep the tissue fluid clear of disease-causing toxic substances, which makes this a system of utmost importance for our health and wellbeing. Very few doctors, though, refer to it when they speak to their patients about the illness they are suffering from.

Practically every type of cancer is preceded by a major, ongoing condition of lymphatic congestion. Wherever lymph drainage is consistently the most insufficient, cancerous tumors manifest first. If more areas of the body are affected in this way, cancers may develop in multiple places. The lymphatic system works closely with the immune system in keeping the body free of harmful metabolic waste products, toxins, pathogens, noxious material, and cell debris. In addition to poor circulation of the blood, congested lymph ducts and lymph nodes cause an overload of harmful waste matter in the tissue fluid. Subsequently, this normally thin vital fluid becomes increasingly thick (syrupy), thus preventing proper nutrient distribution to the cells, which weakens or damages them. Cell mutation occurs when oxygen, carried by the blood to the cells, is continuously hindered from making its way through to them.

The most pressing question is, "Where does lymph congestion begin?" There may be several answers, but the most important ones relate to bile and diet. Restricted bile secretions in the liver and gallbladder due to accumulated gallstones[18] undermine the stomach's and small intestine's ability to digest food properly. Undigested food is naturally subject to decomposition by destructive intestinal bacteria. This permits substantial amounts of waste matter and poisonous substances, such as the highly carcinogenic (cancer-causing) *amines, cadaverines, putrescines,* and other breakdown products of fermented and putrefied food to seep into the intestinal lymph ducts. Along with undigested fats

---

[18] See the author's book, *The Amazing Liver and Gallbladder Flush,* for details on stones in the liver and gallbladder and how to remove them safely and painlessly through liver flushing.

and proteins these poisons enter the body's largest lymphatic structure, the *thoracic duct* and its base, the *cysterna chyli*. The cysterna chyli is a lymph-dilation (in the shape of a sac or oval pool), situated in front of the first two lumbar vertebrae at the level of the belly button (see **Illustration 2**). It extends itself to other smaller sac-like lymph vessels.

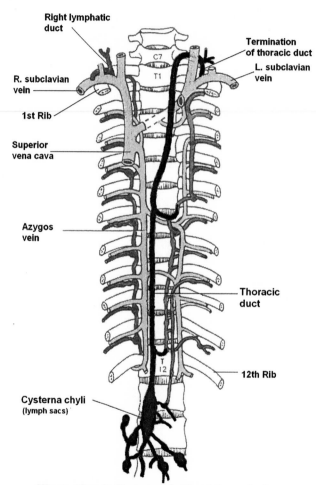

Illustration 2: Cysterna chyli and thoracic duct

Toxins, antigens, and undigested proteins from animal sources, including fish, meat, poultry, eggs, and dairy foods, cause these lymph sacs/pools to become inflamed and to swell (lymphedema). Once the cells of an animal die, which happens seconds after it is killed, cellular enzymes immediately begin to break down their protein structures. The heating/cooking/frying of animal proteins, such as eggs, fish and meat, coagulates (hardens) the proteins and tears apart their natural three-dimensional molecular structure. The resulting so-called "degenerate" proteins are not only useless to the body; they actually become harmful unless they are promptly removed by the lymphatic system. Their presence naturally encourages enhanced microbial activity. Parasites, worms, fungi, and bacteria feed on these pooled wastes. In some cases, allergic reactions occur.

Lymphedema

When lymph congestion exists in the cysterna chyli, this crucial part of the lymphatic system can no longer properly remove the body's worn-out and damaged cell proteins. [Remember, the body has to remove 30 billion old cells each day.] This results in *lymphedema.* You can feel any existing lymphedemas as tender, hard knots by touching or massaging the area of your belly button while lying on your back. These knots are sometimes as large as a fist. Some people describe them as "rocks" in the stomach. These "rocks" are a major cause of middle and low back pain as well as abdominal swelling, bloating and weight gain around the waist area. In fact, they are behind most symptoms of ill health, including heart disease, diabetes, and cancer. Nearly all of the hundreds of cancer patients I have seen suffered from some degree of lymphedema, abdominal distension or bloating. The enlargement of the abdomen is usually accompanied by facial swelling (moon face), a double chin, puffy eyes, and a thickening of the neck—indications of advanced lymphatic congestion.

Many people, who have "grown a tummy," consider this extension of their waist line to be a harmless nuisance or a natural part of aging. They say that almost everyone has an enlarged tummy nowadays, and that this must be normal. They don't realize that they are breeding a living time bomb that may go off some day and injure vital parts of the body. Cancer almost always indicates the existence of such a time bomb.

Eighty percent of the lymphatic system is located at, and associated with, the intestinal tract, therefore making this area of the body the largest center of immune activity. This is no coincidence. The part of the body where most disease-causing agents are combated or generated is, in fact, the intestinal tract. Any lymphedema and other kinds of obstruction in this important part of the lymphatic system are due to an overload of intestinal toxic waste and can lead to potentially serious complications elsewhere in the body.

Wherever a lymph duct is obstructed, an accumulation of lymph exists at a distance to the obstruction. Consequently, the lymph nodes located along such a blocked duct can no longer adequately neutralize or detoxify the following: dead and live phagocytes and their ingested microbes, worn-out tissue cells, cells damaged by disease, products of fermentation, pesticides in food, inhaled or toxic particles, cells from malignant tumors, and many of the millions of cancer cells every healthy person generates each day. Incomplete destruction of these things can cause the lymph nodes to become inflamed, enlarged, and congested with blood. In addition, infected material may enter the bloodstream, causing septic poisoning and acute illnesses. In most cases, though, the lymph blockage occurs gradually over many years, without any "serious" symptoms other than swelling of the abdomen, hands, arms, feet, or ankles or puffiness in the face and eyes. This is often referred to as "fluid retention," a major precursor of chronic illness. Many cancer patients suffer from one or several of these symptoms long before they are diagnosed with a cancerous growth.

Continuous lymphatic obstruction usually leads to cellular mutation. Almost every cancer results from chronic congestion in the cysterna chyli. Eventually, the thoracic duct, which drains the cysterna chyli and carries lymph upward toward the neck into the left lymphatic duct, is overburdened by the constant influx of toxic material and becomes clogged up, too. The thoracic duct connects with numerous other lymphatic ducts (see **Illustrations 2 & 3**) that empty their waste material into the thoracic "sewer canal." Since the thoracic duct has to remove 85% of the body's daily-generated cellular waste and other potentially highly toxic material, a blockage there causes backwashing of waste into other, more distant parts of the body. This results in the swelling that is characteristic of local lymphedema, often found around the ankles.

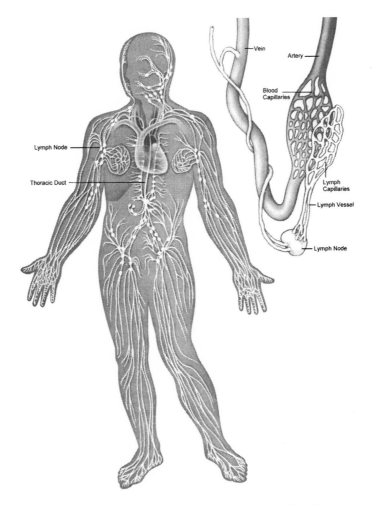

Illustration 3: Lymphatic system and lymph node

When the daily-generated metabolic waste and cellular debris remain trapped in an area of the body for some time, symptoms of disease start manifesting. The trapped waste can eventually become a trigger for abnormal cell growth. The following are but a few typical examples of illness indicators that result directly from chronic, localized lymph congestion:

Obesity, cysts in the uterus or ovaries, enlargement of the prostate gland, rheumatism in the joints, enlargement of the left half of the heart, congestive heart failure, congested bronchi and lungs, enlargement of the neck area, stiffness in the neck and shoulders, backaches, headaches, migraines, dizziness, vertigo, ringing in the ears, earaches, deafness, dandruff, frequent colds, sinusitis, hay fever, certain types of asthma, thyroid enlargement, eye diseases, poor vision, swelling in the breasts, breast lumps, kidney problems, lower back pains, swelling of the legs and ankles, scoliosis, brain disorders, memory loss, stomach trouble, enlarged spleen, irritable bowel syndrome, hernia, polyps in the colon, disorders of the reproductive system, and many more.

If any of these symptoms or a combination thereof persists for a number of years, cancer becomes a distinct possibility.

After collecting the lymph from all parts of the body, except the right side of the head and neck, right arm, and upper right quadrant of the body, it joins the left lymphatic duct. This duct returns the lymph to the circulatory system by draining into the left *subclavian vein* at the root of the neck. This vein enters the *superior vena cava*, which leads straight into the heart. In addition to blocking proper lymph drainage from these various organs or parts of the body, any congestion in the cysterna chyli and thoracic duct causes toxic materials to enter the heart and its arteries. This unduly stresses the heart, possibly enlarging it and causing irregular heartbeat and other complications. It also allows these toxins and disease-causing agents to enter the general circulation and spread to other parts of the body.

To emphasize once more, rarely is there a disease, including cancer, that is not due to lymphatic obstruction. It makes sense that if the main sewer pipe draining wastes from your home becomes clogged up, then all the smaller pipes draining the toilets, sinks, showers, and bathtubs will get clogged up, too, and cause flooding. The obesity epidemic in the USA is largely due to (although not ultimately caused by) congested lymph systems that prevent bodily waste from being eliminated.

Lymph blockage, in the vast majority of cases, has its origin in a congested liver[19] and a detrimental diet and lifestyle. In the extreme eventuality, lymphoma or cancer of the lymph may result, of which Hodgkin's disease is the most common type.

Disease is naturally absent when blood and lymph flow is unhindered and normal. Both types of problems, circulatory and lymphatic, can be successfully eliminated through a series of liver cleanses and by following a balanced diet and lifestyle.

4. Chronic Digestive Problems

Prior to experiencing chronic lymph congestion, a person must have long-term difficulty with digesting food. Improperly digested foods become a breeding place for carcinogens—toxic compounds that can affect cellular behavior.

Four main activities take place in the alimentary tract of our digestive system: *ingestion, digestion, absorption, and elimination.* The alimentary canal begins at the mouth, passes through the thorax, abdomen, and pelvic region, and ends at the anus. When food is *ingested,* a series of digestive processes begin to take place. These can be divided into the *mechanical breakdown* of food through mastication (chewing) and the *chemical breakdown* of food through enzymes. These enzymes are present in the secretions produced by the glands of the digestive system.

Enzymes are minute chemical substances that cause or speed up chemical changes in other substances without themselves being changed. Digestive enzymes are contained in the saliva of the salivary glands of the mouth, the gastric juice in the stomach, the intestinal juice in the small intestine, the pancreatic juice in the pancreas, and the bile in the liver. **It is important to know that digestive and metabolic enzymes (only those produced by the body itself) possess the most powerful anti-cancer properties of any substance in the body. Not producing enough of these enzymes has a direct detrimental effect on cell health and can be considered directly responsible for**

---

[19] The causes of gallstones in the liver are fully discussed in the author's book, *The Amazing Liver and Gallbladder Flush.*

71

cancerous growth in the body, regardless of the location.

Absorption is the process by which tiny nutrient particles of digested food pass through the intestinal walls into the blood and lymph vessels for distribution to the cells of the body. The bowels *eliminate* as feces whatever food substances cannot be digested or absorbed. Fecal matter also contains bile, which carries the waste products that result from the breakdown (catabolism) of red blood cells and other harmful substances. In addition, one third of the excreted waste consists of intestinal bacteria. The body can only function smoothly and efficiently if the bowel removes the daily accumulated waste every day. Intestinal congestion arises when foods are inadequately digested. The natural consequence is the back-flushing of waste into the lymph, blood, and upper parts of the body, including the stomach, chest, throat, neck, sensory organs, and brain.

Health is the natural result of a balanced functioning of each of these major activities in the digestive system.[20] On the other hand, cancer and many similar survival attempts arise whenever one or more of these functions is impaired. The presence of gallstones in the liver and gallbladder has a strong disruptive influence on the digestion and absorption of food, as well as on the elimination of waste.

5. Liver Bile Duct Obstruction

Gallstones are not only found in the gallbladder, but also in the bile ducts of the liver. (Johns Hopkins University refers to them as intrahepatic stones.) In fact, most gallstones are actually formed in the liver, and comparatively few occur in the gallbladder. An estimated 20% of the world's population will develop gallstones in their *gallbladder* at some stage in their lives. This figure, however, does not account for the many more people who will develop gallstones in their *liver* or who already have them. During thirty years of practicing natural medicine, I have dealt

---

[20] How to fully restore all these functions of the digestive system is discussed in detail in the author's book, *Timeless Secrets of Health and Rejuvenation* (www.ener-chi.com).

with thousands of people suffering from all types of diseases. I can document that each person, without exception, has had considerable quantities of gallstones in their liver. Cancer patients and those suffering from arthritis, heart disease, liver disease, and other chronic illnesses, appear to have the most stones in their liver. Surprisingly, only a relative few of them report a history of gallstones in their gallbladder. Gallstones in the liver are the main impediment to acquiring and maintaining good health, youthfulness, and vitality. They are, indeed, one of the major reasons people become ill and have difficulty recuperating from illness, including cancer.

The liver has direct control over the growth and functioning of every cell in the body. Any kind of malfunction, deficiency, or abnormal growth pattern of the cells largely results from poor liver performance. Due to its extraordinary design, the liver often "seems" to perform normally, with a blood test indicating balanced amounts of liver enzymes, even after it has lost up to 60% of its original efficiency. As deceiving as this may be to patient and doctor alike, the origin of most diseases can easily be traced to the liver.[21]

All diseases or symptoms of ill health are caused by an obstruction of some sort. If a blood vessel is blocked and, therefore, can no longer provide speedy delivery of vital oxygen or nutrients to a group of cells, the cells will have to enforce specific emergency measures in order to survive. Of course, many of the afflicted cells will not survive the "famine" and will simply die off. However, other more resilient cells will learn to adjust to the adverse situation, by means of cell mutation, and will feed off trapped, toxic metabolic waste products and everything else they can grab from other cells. Although, in reality, such a survival response helps to prevent the body's immediate demise through possible septic poisoning and organ failure, we tend to label this as "disease." In the case of cell mutation, cancer is the label that is applied.

Cleansing the liver and gallbladder from all accumulated stones helps to restore homeostasis, balance weight, and set the

---

[21] See details in The *Amazing Liver and Gallbladder Flush,* by the author.

precondition for the body to heal itself. The liver cleanse is also one of the best precautions you can take to protect yourself against illness in the future.

Unnatural Foods and Beverages

In the United States, the food industry produces over 40,000 different food products, the vast majority of which have no or very limited nutritional value. Highly processed, refined, "improved," fortified, preserved, flavored, pre-cooked, genetically modified, gassed, radiated, microwave-heated, and other altered foods have the common effect of starving human cells.

Cancer is the result of progressive famine on the cellular level. It occurs when the body no longer receives what it needs to grow according to its original design. To survive and prevent the organs from collapsing due to severe malnutrition and energy depletion, the cell nucleus is left with no other choice but to mutate and begin to function anaerobically.

An anaerobic cell is like a sick, homeless person who, alienated from the rest of society, lives off the decomposed and toxic foods that the affluent, healthy members of society have left behind as garbage. The nutritional value of the typical modern diet is nothing short of useless trash. Take for example, French fries or potato chips. Although they are well known to contain carcinogenic fats and harmful additives/preservatives, millions of American children and adults consume them day after day in large quantities.

Do the following experiment: The next time you order French fries at McDonald's or a similar fast food restaurant, take some of them home with you, and leave them in an open space. You will discover that they will not decompose or even change color (unlike French fries made from fresh potatoes which will quickly shrivel up, turn grey and become moldy). Now, repeat the experiment with a hamburger. The hamburger will also last for years without deterioration. No bacteria will even try to decompose it. These and most other manufactured "foods" such as margarine, for example, are made to last forever, perfectly preserved so they can make it through the lengthy manufacturing and transportation process, and are "safe" for the consumer. Are you wondering what kind of chemicals these foods must be saturated with to enable them to resist even bacteria and mold? Few consumers understand what exactly goes into them, although some of the preservatives are listed on the food labels (but often too small to read). And what can the body possibly do to digest them? Nothing at all. If you are fortunate, they simply pass through the intestinal tract without being digested (diarrhea); it's more likely, though, that they have constipating effects and accumulate in the gut, as seen in the grossly extended tummies of those who eat such Frankenstein foods on a regular basis. Since ingesting these foods causes severe nutritional deficiencies, they also cause food cravings that can never be satisfied. The food industry knows this "dirty little secret" and meets the ever-increasing demand for such "smart" foods by producing an even greater variety of mouth-watering products that especially cater to the obese or overweight. Eye-catching phrases include low cholesterol, fat free, low sodium, low calorie, sugar-free. Although these foods should be utterly unappealing to the taste buds, chemical food additives and flavors ensure they taste great. There are now thousands of different manufactured foods that fall into this category. Of course, the food labels contain no warnings that these chemicals are known carcinogens.

The masses are brainwashed to the point that they believe if an American grocery store or restaurant offers a particular food, it must be good and safe. Just take a moment to learn about the research done on microwave-cooked foods.[22] Why would Russia have banned microwave ovens for several decades if they were harmless? Russian researchers have found decreased nutritional value, cancer-making compounds and brain-damaging radiolytics in virtually all microwave-prepared foods. Eating microwave-prepared meals can also cause loss of memory and concentration, emotional instability and a decline in intelligence, according to the research. The Russian scientists also found decreased nutritional value—or significant dimming of their "vital energy

---

[22] For detailed information, see *Timeless Secrets of Health and Rejuvenation.*

field"—in up to 90 percent of all microwave-prepared foods.

In addition, the B complex, C and E vitamins linked with stress-reduction and the prevention of cancer and heart disease, as well as the essential trace minerals needed for optimum brain and body functioning, were all rendered useless by microwaves, even at short cooking durations. Microwave-cooked food is basically reduced to the nutritional equivalent of cardboard. If you don't want to develop nutrient deficiencies (which is a leading cause of cancer), you may be better off throwing this appliance out of your kitchen. The radiation has been found to accumulate in the kitchen furniture, becoming a constant source of radiation in itself.

Microwave usage in the preparation of food has been found to lead to lymphatic disorders and an inability to protect the body against certain cancers. The research found increased rates of cancer cell formation in the blood of people eating microwave-cooked meals. The Russians also reported increased rates of stomach and intestinal cancers, as well as digestive and excretive disorders, plus a higher percentage of cell tumors, including sarcoma.

Microwaves rip apart the molecular bonds that make food "food." Microwave ovens hurl high-frequency microwaves at food. These boil the moisture within food and its packaging by whipsawing water molecules dizzyingly back-and-forth at more than a billion reversals per second. This frantic friction fractures food molecules, rearranging their chemical composition into weird new configurations unrecognizable as food by human bodies. By destroying the molecular structures of food, the body cannot help but turn the food into waste, but not harmless waste, rather, "nuclear waste."

The Russians have done more research on microwaves than any other nation in the world. By contrast, in the U.S., microwave ovens were introduced to the masses without doing any research on their safety. They now are used almost daily in over 95% of households and many restaurants.

Fortunately, the use of microwaves in cooking, cell phones and other wireless devices is now increasingly being recognized to cause cancer and brain damage, among other serious side effects. (See *Cell Phones and Other Wireless Devices* below.)

Health agencies set up by the government to keep people out of harm's way have their own sinister agendas in allowing deadly drugs and technologies to be marketed on a massive scale. How many people are questioning the FDA as to why it allowed genetically engineered canola oil to sweep the American food and restaurant industry without prior testing? Public records show that the FDA knew about the Canadian research that showed mice fed with this oil developed fatal brain tumors. But the agency was not willing to give up the millions of dollars in "licensing fees" that the approval of canola oil brought with it. Likewise, poisonous drugs like aspartame, Splenda, and MSG are now hidden in the majority of the nation's bestselling manufactured foods and beverages because of the FDA approval. These drugs are more addictive than heroin, caffeine, and nicotine taken together. They make it nearly impossible for their "victims" to abstain from overeating. Their disastrous effects on the human body are well documented, and the FDA, the Centers for Disease Control and Prevention (CDC), and food industry have known about it for many years.

The food industry has only one incentive: to make people consume more food. By placing these addictive drugs into the most popular foods and beverages, the food industry has created a society where the eating habits of the majority of its members have spun out of control. With 75% of the population now overweight or obese, American society as a whole is afflicted by a "tumor" of massive proportions; the resultant ill health of the majority and the skyrocketing medical costs go along with it. This tumor eats up an ever-increasing portion of our national resources. In 2007, $2.3 trillion was spent on healthcare; that's 4.3 times the amount spent on national defense. No other nation in the world spends 16 percent of its gross domestic product (GDP) on healthcare like the U.S. does, and I may add, without any obvious benefits. In fact there is no other society in the world with as many sick people as in the U.S.

Given the purely symptom-oriented approaches to dealing with the most serious disorders today, as you would expect, healthcare costs are spiraling out of control. In fact, these ever-increasing health expenditures now pose the greatest threat to the survival of the economy. Even some of the largest corporations can no longer afford to pay for their sick employees' medical insurance while expanding their businesses at the same time. Just like the US at large, they borrow money to keep their companies afloat. Many are cutting back on their work force, and the employees with the worst health records are the first to go.

Having established the fact that leaving the safeguarding of one's health to government agencies is a foolhardy approach, let us return to the core problem in any serious health crisis, cellular starvation. The cells of the body are not interested in utilizing anything that does not serve their growth. The carcinogenic grease of refined and overheated fats and oils, coloring agents, chemical additives, preservatives, pesticides, and all such unnatural substances, ends up plastering the cells' membranes with impenetrable layers of gunk. This does not even include the billions of poison-filled nutritional supplements Americans consume each day, as if they were real food. Just think of how many vitamin pills the average American swallows day after day, year after year—pills that are loaded with binders, fillers, artificial colors, aspartame, or other deadly sweeteners, to name just a few. If you had the chance to look at a microscopic picture of the cell of a newborn baby, you would see how transparent, thin, and clean the cell membrane is. On the other hand, if you were to examine the cell membranes of a 65-year person eating the typical American diet and being on medication for one ailment or another, you would find these to be dark, thick, and distorted. It doesn't take much to turn such cells into cancer cells.

The cells of a malignant tumor are surrounded by a layer of fibrin[23] that is 15 times thicker than that which surrounds healthy cells. All cancer cells are damaged or wounded. The fibrin coating protects cancer cells against deadly phagocytes, killer lymphocytes, and cytokines.

---

[23] Fibrin is involved in the clotting of blood. It is a fibrillar protein that is polymerized to form a "mesh" that forms a haemostatic plug or clot over a wound site. Recent research has shown that fibrin plays a key role in the inflammatory response and development of rheumatoid arthritis.

Naturally, cells that are compromised in this way are separated from their "community," that is, from all the other cells in the body. These alienated cells are truly "homeless." Homeless cells seem to be out of control, and so doctors attack them with lethal weapons designed to poison, cut or burn them. Their goal is to wipe them out, and they may not realize the serious consequences that attacking cancer cells can have on the surrounding colonies of cells. Those who do realize the probable damage to healthy cells, may feel this is a risk they must take in order to kill the offending cells.

Doctors practically play "Russian roulette" with the lives of their patients when they put them on chemotherapy and/or radiation treatments. They can never predict or know whether the patient will survive the assault or die from it. Dimitris, a Greek medical doctor who had studied and practiced medicine in the U.S. for several years before returning to his native country, came to visit me in Cyprus to see if I could do something for his terminal liver cancer. During the following six months he dealt with and removed all the possible root causes of his cancer, and subsequently the liver tumor had shrunk from the size of an egg to a tiny speck. One day, a former colleague of his convinced him to take one course of the latest and most powerful chemotherapy drug that had just been approved for treatment by the FDA. Dimitris became convinced that killing the last few cancer cells would guarantee the cancer would not return, and so he flew to the U.S. for treatment. Three days later, he was flown back to Greece, inside a coffin. He had died from drug poisoning. I had warned him that when the body goes into a rapid healing mode as he did, stopping this process with poisonous drugs could be fatal. During the healing phase, the body is many times more vulnerable to chemical poisoning than it is in the protection mode, which in this case is represented by a growing cancerous tumor. I have witnessed the same phenomenon in other cancer patients who also gave into the temptation of "finishing off" their last bits of cancer. Their decision turned out to be a fatal one.

It is extremely difficult for the body to protect itself against poisoning when it is trying to heal itself. To damage healthy cells in the process of destroying cancer cells through chemotherapy drugs or radiation is bound to breed new, more aggressive cancer cells. The only real chance of surviving cancer depends on the amount of support the patient musters to strengthen the body's own healing efforts.

The approach to treating cancer as a disease is not only fraught with dangers and needless suffering, but it also fails to address the underlying issue of diet. By feeding our children and ourselves non-physiological foods, such as mold-resistant French fries and hamburgers, that thicken cell membranes and force cells to mutate in order to function in an anaerobic environment, we are creating diseases that will literally wipe out entire communities; and this trend has already begun to take its course.

Our modern society suffers greatly from cancer. It is up to each one of us to make those choices that favor life over death. What we put in our mouth has a lot to do with how our society will survive. Considering the statistic that one in every two Americans will develop some form of cancer, and knowing that the prospects of avoiding cancer are worsening each year, it only makes sense that we stay away from manufactured foods (and other cancer-producing factors) as much as possible. If you have cancer, your chances of recovery will increase dramatically when you eat only natural foods that have not been manipulated or altered by the food industry. I especially recommend that you consume only organically grown foods, ideally locally grown, during the recovery period. This allows the body to focus on healing rather than forcing it to engage its already battered immune system in battles with chemical additives and pesticides.

Changing your diet greatly reduces your risk of developing cancer. Diet also plays a critical role in bringing about a permanent remission if cancer has already occurred. In an estimated 60% or more of all malignant cancers, diet plays a leading role in its onset. An anti-cancer diet can effectively cut your cancer risk by two-thirds. The most successful cancer-preventing diet is still the vegetarian model.

Compelling demonstrations of how entire countries can be virtually cancer-free are provided in population studies. Thus far, over 200 studies have been done on cancer occurrence among different groups of people in the world. As it turns out, cancer rates are much lower in developing nations than in the U.S. The average American diet, consisting of very fatty, protein-rich, highly processed food items, has almost nothing in common with the diet typically consumed by folks in developing countries. Fruits, vegetables, legumes, and grains still form the standard diet of people living in most developing countries, although the Western influence of bringing unnatural and fast foods into their towns and villages is now making its way into the eating habits of these populations. With these newly introduced, and now "fashionable" eating habits, formerly unheard of disorders like osteoporosis, skin cancer, heart disease, arthritis, and other problems are becoming more and more common in their larger cities.

To save our nation from self-destruction, we have no option but to return to the foods that nature has designed for us to eat. This also means we need to avoid foods that nature does not create. No natural contract exists between our bodies and margarine, for example. Margarine is a laboratory "food" that a natural organism is not equipped to make use of. It is just one molecule away from plastic! Just leave margarine somewhere in a warm, dark, moist environment where bacteria are plentiful, and you will discover that these bacteria will leave it alone. They treat this unnatural product as if it were actually plastic.

For millions of years, the human body relied for its sustenance on natural foods that grew around it, and so it is delusional to believe that our bodies can suddenly learn to subsist on the barrage of new, manufactured foods that have flooded our food markets and grocery stores. We don't even know whether a food, such as corn, soybean products, potatoes, is man-made (genetically engineered) or not. Most manufactured foods contain some genetically modified food ingredients. In truth, food that is not grown by nature, cannot serve as food at all. The body has no connection to or recognition of man-made foods that no longer match the "signature" of real foods. Instead of nourishing the cells of the body, manufactured foods slowly starve them to death by accumulating in the organs and tissues. **Thus, feeding the body exclusively with manufactured foods is simply suicidal. Eating the more or less typical American diet consisting of**

red meat, fried foods, full-fat dairy products, refined grains, and desserts is, in fact, synonymous with unintentionally killing oneself.

In an observational study, investigators examined the relationship between the dietary patterns of more than 1,000 people who had been treated for stage III colon cancer and their risk of colon cancer recurrence. The researchers found that those who followed a typical American diet were three times more likely to experience a recurrence of colon cancer than their counterparts who followed a mostly vegetarian diet, and they also were more likely to die. The study, which was reported in the *Journal of the American Medical Association,* is the first to address the effect of diet on recurrence in a population of colon cancer survivors. The researchers say, the results strongly suggest that a diet consisting primarily of red and processed meats, French fries, refined grains, and sweets and desserts increases the risk of cancer recurrence and decreases survival.

There is some good news, though, that certain foods can somewhat counteract the cancer-producing effects of the typical American diet. A Japanese study at Nagoya University showed that the pigment in purple corn impedes the development of cancer in the colon. The researchers divided animals into two groups, one of which received food mixed with a natural carcinogenic substance found in the charred parts of roasted meat and fish, and another group that also received 5% pigment of purple corn. In the group that was fed the carcinogen, 85% developed colon caner, compared with only 40% that also received the pigment. Other studies showed that purple corn also prevents obesity and diabetes.

Deadly Cell Phones and Other Wireless Devices

An increasing number of medical researchers, environment protection agencies, governments and individuals are concerned that wireless technology may be causing serious harm to people and the environment:

- The country of Germany has recently (2007) warned the population to avoid wireless devices.
- In September 2007, based on its analysis of research conducted in 15 different laboratories, the EU's European Environment Agency (EEA) issued warnings to all European citizens advising them to stop using Wi-Fi and cell phones, citing fears that the ever-present use of wireless technology has the potential to become the next public health disaster on the level of tobacco smoking, asbestos, and lead in automobile gas (as reported by The BioInitiative Working Group).
- The Israeli government recently banned the placement of antennas used for cell phone reception on residential buildings.
- As reported on CBC (July 12, 2008), Toronto's department of public health has advised teenagers and young children to limit their use of cell phones, in order to avoid potential health risks. According to the advisory, which is the first of its kind in Canada, children under the age of eight should only use a cell phone in emergencies, and teenagers should limit calls to less than 10 minutes.
- As little as 10 minutes on a cell phone can trigger changes in brain cells linked to cell division and cancer, suggests a new study conducted by researchers from the Weizmann Institute of Science in Israel and published in the *Biochemical Journal*. The changes they observed were not caused by the heating of tissues.
- Regular cell phone use raises the risk of developing a brain tumor for many users, according to a new Finnish study published online in the *International Journal of Cancer*. The study, conducted by numerous researchers from many universities, found firm corollary evidence that using a cell phone causes the risk of getting a brain tumor called a glioma to rise

by 40 to 270[24] percent on the side of the head preferred for using the phones. This is the same type of brain tumor doctors discovered in Ted Kennedy. Malignant glioma is the most common primary brain tumor, accounting for more than half of the 18,000 primary malignant brain tumors diagnosed each year in the United States, according to the National Cancer Institute.

- Prolonged cell phone use may damage sperm in male users, suggests a study by researchers at the Cleveland Clinic Lerner College of Medicine at Case Western Reserve University in Ohio. The discovery was made during an ongoing study of 51,000 male health professionals in the United States.
- Pregnant mothers, who use cell phones 2-3 times per day, are found to give birth to children with malfunctioning cells. Also young children exposed to cell phone radiation are found to develop serious growth problems.

The media industry is the largest and most lucrative industry in the world, much bigger than oil. Almost every significant company is run, owned or heavily influenced by the 5 - 6 media giants. Cell phones make up a huge junk of that. Any attempt to blame cell phones for the massive increase of cancers in the world is ridiculed and squashed, just like cigarette smoking was not too long ago. Some people are okay with waiting until finally there is solid "evidence" that radio waves can cause cancer before they give up their beloved cell phones. Others continue using them just as many continue smoking, although the risks for the latter are known. It is really up to each individual to decide what to do about it. For me, personally, there is no question about it. I detect harmful energies from a distance, and certainly when they come as close to my body as a cell phone does. I use my cell phone very rarely, and if I do, it's just for a minute or two. I never felt comfortable with them, long before research began to indicate that they are not harmless at all.

---

[24] Those who used modern cellular phones for more than 2,000 hours in their lifetime had the highest risk increase. Surprisingly, the risk was highest among people under the age of 20.

On a different note, certain U.S. states and countries in Europe are banning the use of cell phones while driving. In England, where cell phone use is prohibited while driving, they are about to implement a new law that prohibits the use of hands-free phones as well. The government found that such phone use disorients the driver and increases the risk of accidents. The disorientation lasts for up to 10 minutes after use. In comparison, a conversation with another person in the car showed no such adverse effects. This may indicate that it is not the conversation (using hands-free car phones) that interferes with concentration, reaction and focused attention, but rather the brain's exposure to harmful rays. You are still exposed to these rays 2 to 3 feet away from you. The other explanation is that speaking to another person who is not physically present requires your brain to create an image of that person in your mind. Since the brain cannot compute and sustain two visuals at the same time, disorientation results. In other words, you can no longer focus on your driving and you may not react as readily, especially in situations of heavy traffic. Holding a phone to your ear also restricts your peripheral vision, and you may not be able to see a car that is coming toward you from the side.

Most users of cell phones and other wireless devices have no idea what low radiation can do to them, since it isn't tangible and only very few sensitive people experience a negative effect from them. Only when you stand in front of a radar device will you start perspiring/cooking from the inside out, just like food being cooked in the microwave oven. The heat is generated by the rapid movement of molecules (friction) and the breaking down of molecular bonds. Each year, millions of birds are killed when they get too close to, or sit on, cell towers. And apparently, the same can happen to the human body when it is exposed to this type of radiation on a regular basis. After all, human cells are made of molecules and molecular bonds are broken and destroyed when exposed to radiation. Strong radiation can literally burn off the entire skin of a person from the inside out. Weak radiation does this more slowly and less dramatically. But as you may know, X-rays, CT-scans radiation and microwaves accumulate, and you can never tell when the body responds with a healing crisis, such as cancer.

Many people are very unsuspecting, unconcerned or naive with regard to their health. The incidence of chronic disease has moved from 10% to 90% in just 100 years. It may not be just one thing that causes these degenerative diseases, but a combination of factors. But yes, each factor becomes significant when combined with others.

Everyone must make their own choices and decide what's good for them and what isn't. There is no point trying to persuade someone, for this can cause resentment, a much more serious cause of illness than radio waves or cigarette smoking.

I am currently researching a simple device that can protect the body from the harmful rays and electromagnetic fields that almost constantly surround and bombard us (e.g. cars, computers, cell phones, electric appliances, cell towers, fluorescent lights, harmful chemicals in foods and the environments, and other common stress factors). The device works instantly, and it may have enormous implications for the health and wellbeing of individuals and families. In the past 12 years I have tested nearly a dozen methods or devices that supposedly protect against cell phone radiation, with disappointing results. However, I am extremely exited about this one. Soon I will have completed my research and will post details on my web site.

The EM-Heavy Metal Connection

In 1993, the cell phone industry and U.S. government agencies gave the well known American researcher, Dr. George Louis Carlo, a $28 million research grant to put to rest, once and for all, any concerns about risks associated with cell phones. Much to the benefit and relief of the industry, initial results covering three years of research indicated that there were no problems with cell phone use. However, by 1999, Dr. Carlo had gained significantly more evidence indicating a risk to DNA, eye cancers, and brain tumors.

Following the discovery that cell phones can cause serious health conditions, including cancer, Carlo developed a theory that low frequency cell phone signals interfere with normal cell function. He found that cells exposed to cell phone radiation caused them to go into a protective/defensive mode—similar to what occurs during the "fight or flight response"—which prevents movement of nutrients and waste products through the cellular membrane. The inability to absorb nutrients weakens, damages, or kills cells; and not being able to remove wastes outside cells results in a buildup of toxins. This observation led Carlo to believe there was a close connection between the massive upsurge in usage of wireless technology and the dramatic increase in autism. He hypothesized that young children exposed to electromagnetic (EM) radiation are less able to process heavy metals ingested through air, food and water, and as a result, begin to accumulate these in their tissues. If this happens to be the brain tissue, it causes neurological damage, including autism. In older people, such an accumulation of heavy metals in the brain can lead to damage of the DNA, multiple sclerosis and Alzheimer's disease. Mercury is already toxic at one in one billion-part quantities. That is about the same concentration of one grain of salt in one swimming pool.

It is a well established fact that mercury and other heavy metals such as lead are linked with neurological disorders like autism. In 2003, the *International Journal of Toxicology* released a study that showed the hair of autistic babies contained significantly less mercury and other heavy metals. Autistic babies are not able to excrete the toxic metals via the hair and the body's other natural waste removal outlets (hair is a waste product containing excessive proteins and minerals, among other things). Hence, these toxic metals remain trapped in their brains.

To prove the theory that EM radiation prevents autistic children from releasing toxic metals, Carlo and his colleague, Tamara Mariea, set up a trial with 20 autistic children. The study was reported in the November 2007 issue of the *Journal of the Australian College of Nutrition and Environmental Medicine*. The children spent a minimum of four hours, two or three times a week, in a clinic that was completely EM-free. They received no other treatment. Within three months, the children started to excrete heavy metals from their bodies.

If in fact EM radiation inhibits metal elimination from the body, then regular cell phone use can be blamed for increasing the chances of developing cancer. Many trace metals undermine the functions of a huge range of enzymes and proteins involved in cell signaling, life cycles, replication, and cell death. Metals such as cadmium are known to be aggressively mutagenic, damaging DNA, and elevated concentrations in the body have been linked to prostate, renal and lung cancers. Similarly, raised levels of lead have been associated with myeloma (a cancer of plasma cells) and leukemia, as well as cancers of the stomach, small intestine, large intestine, ovary, kidney, and lung.

Other metals, including chromium and zinc, have been associated with the more rapid progression of breast, colon, rectal, ovarian, lung, bladder and pancreatic cancers, and leukemia. Also nickel, antimony and cobalt are considered to be mutagens and have been linked to lung and nasal cancer.

Note: See Chapter Five on how about harmful radiation, pesticides and heavy metal poisoning.

What has Gum Disease to do With It?

When researchers looked at data collected between 1986 and 2002, they found that men with gum disease had a 63 percent higher chance of getting pancreatic cancer, even if they'd never smoked. Scientists are not exactly sure why gum disease and cancer are linked, but some theorize gum disease can increase inflammation that can be spread throughout the body. Other research has already linked gum disease to various diseases as well, including heart disease, stroke, diabetes, respiratory issues and lung infections.

American forefathers used brine to preserve their food and kill bacteria. The same germ-removing action of salt water can be harnessed to keep the gums free of infection. Millions of people have used warm salt water rinses to cure oral abscesses, gum boils, etc. Apparently, the warm salt water helps to draw excessive toxic fluid out of the gum tissue, thereby reducing swelling, alleviating pain, and killing harmful bacteria. This allows the gums to heal and keep the teeth healthy, too. If used in an irrigating device, the warm salt water reaches all gum line crevices and periodontal pockets, which is important for complete reversal of gum disease and tooth decay.

Rinsing or irrigating the mouth with salt water several times a day is usually enough to prevent and reverse gum disease. For situations of advanced gum disease, however, you may also use *Sanguinary*, an herbal extract, which has been used as a mouth rinse for centuries by native cultures.

Gum disease indicates the presence of large amounts of toxins in the body, especially in the alimentary canal which begins in the mouth and ends in the anus. In addition to the above rinsing procedures, it is also important to address the underlying causes, such as poor diet, dehydration, irregular lifestyle, congested liver and intestinal tract, and emotional stress.

Soladey's Dental Solution

I personally use a *Soladey* toothbrush to clean my teeth. Soladey has a patented design that is scientifically and clinically proven to significantly eliminate plaque more effectively than your regular toothbrush, without the use of toothpaste or dental floss. Soladey features a titanium oxide (TIO2) metal rod, which is sensitive to light. It creates a natural ionic chemical reaction that separates the plaque from your teeth enamel and removes tobacco, coffee and other stains using the natural attraction of ions. You might have heard of a room ionizer that also produces ions. Plaque contains particles with a positive charge (positive ions). When the titanium rod reacts with light, it creates negative ions that attract the positive ions, like a magnet. The plaque just disintegrates and falls off your teeth, washing away when your rinse. Other stains are sucked right out of your teeth using this process.

There have been four clinical trials at four different dental universities in Canada and Japan, and they all found that the people who used Soladey had significantly less plaque on their teeth compared to the people who used the ordinary brush. The research also showed an improvement in gingivitis. So Soladey works to protect your gums—as well as reduce plaque.

The scientific principles behind Soladey have been around since the 1970s and Soladey has now been sold in Japan for a few years—where it sells two million brush units and five million replacement heads every year. Clinical studies on the effectiveness of Soladey technology to remove dental plaque have been conducted at Osaka Dental University, Nippon Dental University, Nihon University and the University of Saskatchewan in Canada. All institutions certify that Soladey was more effective in the removal of plaque and whitening of dental enamel than any regular bristle toothbrush on the market today. (See *Product Information* or visit www.ener-chi.com/soladey.htm.)

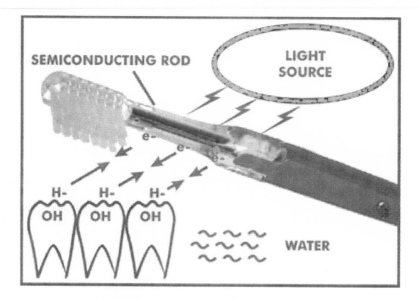

Illustration 4: Soladey toothbrush in action

Sunglasses and Sunscreens— A Major Cause of Cancer

Unfortunately, the ultraviolet portion of sunlight is the most easily eliminated by windows, houses, spectacles, sunglasses, sun lotions, and clothing. And why is that a bad thing? Because ultraviolet light constitutes one of the most powerful natural medicines the world has ever seen. By the year 1933, researchers found there were over 165 different diseases for which sunlight proved to be a beneficial treatment, including tuberculosis, hypertension, diabetes, and almost every type of cancer. To this day, no other treatment has shown such a wide range of benefits as sunlight.

The miraculous complete cures of tuberculosis and many other diseases facilitated by doctors in the early twentieth century made headlines at the time. Remarkably, though, the sun's healing rays remained ineffective if the patients wore sunglasses. Sunglasses block out important rays of the light spectrum which the body requires for essential biological functions. Today, for whatever sinister reasons, the population is being bombarded with warnings about sunbathing and the risks of skin cancer.

The sun is now considered the main culprit for causing skin cancer, certain cataracts leading to blindness, and aging of the skin. Only those who take the "risk" of exposing themselves to sunlight find that the sun actually makes them feel better, provided they don't use sunglasses, sunscreens or burn their skin. The UV rays in sunlight actually stimulate the thyroid gland to increase hormone production, which in turn increases the body's basal metabolic rate. This assists both in weight loss and improved muscle development. Farm animals fatten much faster when kept indoors, and so do people who stay out of the sun. Therefore, if you want to lose weight or increase your muscle tone, expose your body to the sun on a regular basis. Remember, being overweight or obese is major risk factor for developing cancer.

Any person who misses out on sunlight becomes weak and suffers mental and physical problems as a result. His vital energy diminishes in due time, which is reflected in his quality of life. The populations in Northern European countries like Norway and Finland, which experience months of darkness every year, have a higher incidence of irritability, fatigue, illness, insomnia, depression, alcoholism, and suicide than those living in the sunny parts of the world. Their skin cancer rates are higher, too. For example, the incidence of *melanoma* (skin cancer) on the Orkney and Shetland Isles, north of Scotland, is 10 times that of Mediterranean islands.

UV light is known to activate an important skin hormone called *solitrol*. Solitrol influences our immune system and many of our body's regulatory centers, and, in conjunction with the pineal hormone *melatonin,* causes changes in mood and daily biological rhythms. *The hemoglobin* in our red blood cells requires ultraviolet (UV) light to bind to the oxygen needed for all cellular functions. Lack of sunlight can, therefore, be held co-responsible for almost any kind of illness, including skin cancer and other forms of cancer. Using sun protection protects only the multi-billion dollar sunscreen and cancer industry but not your skin or your life. Consider these remarkable scientifically proven facts:

Ultraviolet light
- improves electrocardiogram readings
- lowers blood pressure and resting heart rate
- improves cardiac output when needed (not contradictory to lower resting heart rate)
- reduces cholesterol, if required
- increases glycogen stores in the liver
- balances blood sugar
- enhances energy, endurance, and muscular strength
- improves the body's resistance to infections due to an increase of lymphocytes and phagocytic index (the average number of bacteria ingested per leukocyte in the patient's blood)
- controls a gene that is responsible for producing a powerful broad-spectrum antibiotic throughout the body
- enhances the oxygen-carrying capacity of the blood
- increases sex hormones
- improves resistance of the skin to infections

- raises one's tolerance to stress and reduces depression

On the other hand, there is not a single scientific study which can prove that sunlight itself is responsible for causing skin cancers or other illnesses. There are always other factors present, such as acidosis of the tissues (due to eating an overly acidifying diet consisting of animal proteins, trans fatty acids, and manufactured foods and beverages), most pharmaceutical drugs, an accumulation of heavy metals and harmful chemicals in the tissues, toxic blood, a severely congested liver, an unbalanced lifestyle, and foremost of all, sunglasses and sunscreens.

The human body was designed to absorb UV light for very good reasons; otherwise we would have been born with a natural sunscreen for UV light on our skin and in our eyes. One of the most important reasons is that UV radiation is necessary for normal cell division. Lack of sunlight disrupts normal cell growth, which can lead to cancer. Wearing sunglasses, including regular UV-reflecting spectacles and contact lenses, is largely responsible for certain degenerative eye diseases, such as macular degeneration. Most people who wear sunglasses on a regular basis report continuously weakening eyesight.

Depriving your eyes of adequate exposure to ultraviolet light can have serious consequences for your skin and even pose a risk to your life. Normally, as soon as the optic nerves of your eyes sense sunlight, your pituitary gland produces hormones that act as boosters for your *melanocytes*. Melanocytes produce melanin, the pigment that gives skin its natural color and protection against sunburn. When skin is exposed to the sun, melanocytes produce more pigment, causing the skin to tan, or darken, and your melanocytes start producing melanin on overdrive. However, when you wear sunglasses, this process becomes disrupted. Instead of kick-starting the melanocyte production to protect your skin against sunburn, your pituitary gland thinks it is getting dark outside and, thus, it greatly reduces production of melanocyte-stimulating hormones. Subsequently, your skin produces less melanin, which causes it to be less protected and, in turn, become damaged.

The dramatically increased incidence of skin damage

seemingly caused by the sun (but really by wearing sunglasses) is exploited by the sunscreen and cancer industry. The main reason the dermatology industry promotes sunscreen products is because it is heavily funded by sunscreen manufacturers. The pharmaceutical and medical industries never intended to cure diseases. Right from the beginning, it was their intention to make a lot of money by producing drugs and chemicals that would create new diseases for which they would develop specific drugs and procedures to relieve symptoms, but never really eliminate them. In the above example of sunlight, by advertising the dangers of sunlight and promoting the use of sunglasses and sunscreens, the pharma/medical industry made certain that the number of skin cancers and numerous other health problems would increase. They then recommended the appropriate treatments to combat these diseases, which, in turn, will lead to further escalations of these same diseases. These principles of psychological deception are well known to the industry and are applied to almost every so-called disease. The result is that nearly every person in the United States already has or will develop one or several serious illnesses at some stage in their life. Something as "harmless" as sunglasses or sunscreens has created a health disaster of unimaginable proportions.

As the health author of web site *NaturalNews* reported recently, a CDC study shows that 97 percent of Americans are contaminated with an extremely toxic sunscreen chemical called *oxybenzone*. This chemical is found in nearly 600 sunscreen products, including children's formulas. Most sun-blocking creams and lotions also contain *avobenzone* for broad-spectrum protection against short- and long-wave UVA rays which are falsely considered to be the main culprits responsible for long-term skin damage.[25] Most sunscreens also contain a cocktail of a dozen or more cancer-promoting fragrance chemicals and numerous petrochemical-derived synthetic substances. Many of these carcinogenic chemicals are readily absorbed through the

---

[25] For details on how blocking out of some or all UV rays leads to damage of deeper skin tissue, see "Heal Yourself with Sunlight" or Chapter Eight of "*Timeless Secrets of Health and Rejuvenation.*"

skin, much to the annoyance of the consumer who has to keep reapplying the "protective" sunscreens. [Sunscreens come in the form pf lotion, cream, oil, ointment, stick, gel/jelly, spray, liquid, and pad.]

The producers of these products claim that most of the harmful chemicals become degraded in the presence of sunlight and must therefore be safe for the consumer, a claim that is outright false since almost every person in America is contaminated by sunscreen chemicals (according to the U.S. Centers for Disease Control and Prevention). Avobenzone [butyl-methyoxydibenzoylmethane and oxybenzone particularly penetrate the skin very quickly. Other chemicals found in sunscreens include dixoybenzone, PABA and PABA esters (ethyl dihydroxy propyl PAB, glyceryl PABA, p-aminobenzoic acid, padimate-O or octyl dimethyl PABA, Cinnamates (cinoxate, ethylhexyl p-methoxycinnamate, octocrylene, octyl methoxycinnamate), Salicylates (ethylhexyl salicylate, homosalate, octyl salicylate), Digalloyl trioleate and Menthyl anthranilate.

There is an almost complete lack of any adequate safety testing of these chemicals. Cosmetics contain them, too, and the body absorbs them like a sponge.

Many heavily-used chemical sunscreens have a strong free radical generating effect, which is the main reason behind skin cancer. Scientists use such chemicals to start free radical reactions during chemical synthesis. These chemicals are so dangerous that those who handle them in a laboratory must keep them away from their skin. When combined with other chemicals and exposed to ultraviolet light, they then generate the copious amounts of free radicals required to bring about the desired chemical reactions. On your skin, however, such chemical reactions are anything but desirable.

Oxybenzone, for example, which is found in 97% of Americans, is activated by ultraviolet light that breaks its double bond to produce two free radical sites. These free radicals then oxidize and damage fats, proteins, and DNA of the cells—the types of damage that occur in skin aging and the development of skin cancers.

One major study looked at how sunscreens could increase melanoma risk. Its team of researchers, , Cedric F. Garland, et al, found that worldwide, the greatest rise in melanoma has occurred in countries where chemical sunscreens have been heavily promoted by the medical establishment and pharma/chemical industry. Queensland now has more incidences of melanoma per capita than any other place on Earth. The study was published by *American Journal of Public Health*, Vol. 82, No. 4, April 1992, pp. 614-15.

The question why the incidence of skin cancer has increased so dramatically since the massive promotion of sunscreens should have raised a red flag among consumers, but, instead, it made them lather their skin with even more of these deadly chemicals. The mass media (financed largely by drug giants) made certain that the population would not hear about such important studies as the following ones:

Dr. Gordon Ainsleigh in California found that the 17% increase in breast cancer observed between 1981 and 1992 may be the result of the pervasive use of sunscreens over the past decade (Ainsleigh, H. Gordon. Beneficial effects of sun exposure on cancer mortality. *Preventive Medicine*, Vol. 22, February 1993, pp. 132-40).

According to several studies, men who regularly use sunscreens have a higher rate of melanoma, and women using sunscreens have a higher rate of basal cell carcinoma. (Garland, Cedric F., et al. Effect of sunscreens on UV radiation-induced enhancement of melanoma growth. *Journal of the National Cancer Institute*, Vol. 86, No. 10, May 18, 1994, pp. 798-801:Larsen, H.R.

"Sunscreens: do they cause skin cancer." *International Journal of Alternative & Complementary Medicine*, 1994; 12(12): 17-19; Farmer, K.C. & Naylor, M.F.

"Sun exposure, sunscreens, and skin cancer prevention: a year-round concern." Ann Pharmacother, 1996; 30(6):662-73.

The medical industry's biggest argument in favor of using sunscreens is that they prevent skin cancer because they prevent sunburn, implying that skin cancers are caused by sunburn. But this is more a correlation than a cause-effect relationship. More recent studies done in England and Australia actually found much higher skin cancer rates among people who live mostly indoors compared with those who spend most of their time outdoors.

As Drs. Cedric and Frank Garland of the University of California have pointed out, there is no scientific proof that sunscreens protect against melanoma or basal cell carcinoma in humans (Garland, C.F., et al. "Could sunscreens increase melanoma risk?" *American Journal of Public Health*, 1992; 82(4): 614-615.) According to the Garlands, the increased use of chemical sunscreens is the primary cause of the skin cancer epidemic. A study by Drs. Mike Brown (Kate Law of the Cancer Research Campaign) and Philippe Autier (European Institute of Oncology in Milan) reported that children using sunscreen returned from holiday with more skin moles—a possible sign of increased cancer risk. Whether or not sunscreens increase the risk of developing skin cancer, at least there is overwhelming evidence that sunscreens don't prevent skin cancer.

In February 1998, epidemiologist Marianne Berwick of Memorial Sloan-Kettering Cancer Center in New York presented a careful analysis of data on sunscreen use and skin cancer at the annual meeting of the American Association for the Advancement of Science. Sunscreens may not protect against skin cancer, including melanoma, she concluded. "We don't really know whether sunscreens prevent skin cancer," said Dr. Berwick. "After examining the available epidemiological data and conducting our own large case-control population-based study, we have found no relationship between sunscreen use at any age and the development of melanoma skin cancer," said Dr. Berwick. Although sunscreens do prevent sunburn, Dr. Berwick concluded that sunburn itself is not the direct cause of cancer. She argued that if people develop melanoma, it may be because they are genetically susceptible and likely to develop skin cancer regardless of the amount of sunlight exposure or protection from sunscreen.[26] Dr. Berwick objected to the universal blanket advice

[26] For more details about the possible factors responsible for developing skin cancer, see *Heal Yourself with Sunlight* or *Timeless Secrets of Health and Rejuvenation*.

about using sunscreens during all time spent outdoors.

Dr. Berwick's previously conducted research (1996) found no relationship between a history of sunburn and the development of melanoma.

The American Academy of Dermatology (AAD), which is largely funded by advertising sunscreen and skin care products, of course strongly condemned Dr. Berwick's research and called her a "number crunching scientist." I guess that's what scientists do, crunch numbers.

Now back to what sunscreens can actually do to you. They may not only be responsible for melanomas, but for many other types of cancer and dysfunctions as well. What's most disturbing is that many commonly used sunscreen chemicals have strong estrogenic actions which may seriously affect sexual development in children and sexual function in adults, and further increase cancer risks. Exposing your body to chemicals that can alter hormonal balance puts your health at great risk, to put it mildly.

Of course, the sunscreen industry neglects to inform you that there is not much difference between drinking your sunscreen lotion and lathering it on your skin, except ingesting it would actually cause you much less harm because your digestive system would filter out most of the poison. The skin has no other option than to dump this cocktail of carcinogens right into the circulatory system, and from there, into the liver, kidneys, heart and brain. I will leave it to your imagination what such a chemical assault means for these vital organs.

The Vitamin D Factor

Sunglasses and sunscreen agents are among the most health-endangering products that exist because they block absorption of ultraviolet rays which your body needs to produce vitamin D. Besides hindering the essential exposure of your eyes and skin to the rays of the sun, the use of sunscreens and sunglasses is largely responsible for the chronic vitamin D deficiency that plagues 80% of the American population. Vitamin D deficiency is associated with depression, prostate cancer, breast cancer, osteoporosis and almost every other degenerative disorder. "The elderly, who spend little time in the sun and use sunscreen agents frequently, may be at risk for vitamin D deficiency," according to a statement made by the Mayo Clinic. Vitamin D deficiency is strongly associated with bone disease and fracture. Makes you wonder why so many elderly people suffer from bone disorders.

New research findings (published in the *Archives of Internal Medicine,* June 9, 2008; 168(11):1174-1180) join a growing body of evidence indicating that an adequate level of vitamin D, which you can obtain by spending an average of 20 minutes in the sun each day (dark-skinned people may need an hour or more), is crucial to maintaining good health. Men who are deficient in vitamin D were found to have more than double the normal risk of suffering a heart attack or dying even after all other possible risk factors such as hypertension, obesity and high levels of blood fat were excluded. Populations in northern countries (with less intense sunlight and lower levels of vitamin D) have higher incidence of heart disease than sun-filled southern countries. In additon, more heart attacks occur in the winter months, when sunlight is scarce. Furthermore, low levels of vitamin D showed an increased risk of developing diabetes and dying from breast cancer.

A new study conducted by scientists at the German Cancer Research Center Deutsches Krebsforschungszentrum, DKFZ, collaborating with researchers of the University Hospitals in Hamburg-Eppendorf, provides clear evidence that post-menopausal women with low blood levels of vitamin D clearly have a significantly increased risk of breast cancer. The study was released in April 2008 and published in the medical journal *Carcinogenesis.* Among other cancer-inhibiting effects, sunlight-induced vitamin D increases the self-destruction of mutated cells and reduces the spread and reproduction of cancer cells.

Sun exposure can help you to prevent as many as 16 different types of cancer including pancreatic, lung, breast, ovarian, prostate, and colon cancers. Research has clearly shown that it can cut your risk by as much as 60 percent. On the other hand, lack of sun exposure and subsequent vitamin D deficiency kills more than one million people each year.

Comparatively, the risk of being harmed by the sun is minimal. The most dangerous of skin cancers, which is melanoma, usually appears in parts of the skin where the sun does not reach at all, or not reach enough. If you have the opportunity, for optimal protection expose your entire body to the sun, including the private parts.

You Can't be Happy and Healthy Without It—The Serotonin Connection

Medical researchers are growing increasingly excited about a wonder drug that may significantly reduce your risk of heart disease, cancer, diabetes and many other diseases: sunshine. Amazingly, one of nature's best medicines is right outside your doorstep, but many people choose to ignore it. We all know that plants and animals deprived of adequate sunlight become sick. Is it so surprising to find that humans could actually suffer the same fate? After all, the human body was genetically designed to be outdoors most of the time. By contrast, most people in the modernized world spend the majority of their time indoors.

Spending most of the time inside buildings—cut off from the UV light and other healing rays of the sun—creates an enormous challenge for the body, mind and emotions. Ultimately, all hormones in the body are regulated by the circadian rhythm (day and night cycle). The powerful neurotransmitter and intestinal hormone *serotonin* closely follows the "movement" of the sun in respect to the earth. Peak secretion occurs during noon time when the sun's intensity is the strongest.

In the central nervous system, serotonin plays an important role as a neurotransmitter (hormone) in the modulation of anger, depression, aggression, body temperature, mood, sleep, sexuality, appetite, and metabolism. In the gastrointestinal tract, which contains about 90% of the body's total serotonin, it is responsible for balanced digestive functions. In the blood, the major storage site is platelets, which collect serotonin for use in mediating post-injury vasoconstriction. Recent research suggests that serotonin plays an important role in liver regeneration and acts as a mitogen (induces cell division) throughout the body (Wikipedia). Failed induction of cell division is a leading cause of cancer.

In addition, recent Italian research conducted at the European Molecular Biology Laboratory in Monterotondo, Italy found that defective signaling of serotonin in the brain may be at the root cause of *Sudden Infant Death Syndrome* (SIDS). This makes a lot of sense. Newborn babies who are being kept in dark rooms and rarely get out into the sun are deprived of vitamin D (purposefully not supplied by mother's milk) and produce little or no serotonin. Worldwide, many more babies die of SIDS in one year than who die of cancer, heart disease, pneumonia, child abuse, cystic fibrosis and muscular dystrophy combined. The Italian research shows that the tested mice suffered drops in heart rate and other symptoms of SIDS, and many of the animals died at an early age. Low levels of serotonin in the animals' brainstems, which control heartbeat and breathing, may have caused sudden death, researchers said in the July 4, 2008 issue of *Science*. Since serotonin in humans controls about the same functions as in mice, researchers believe that the same phenomenon occurs in human infants.

The implications of all the existing research conducted on serotonin are wide-reaching. Any prolonged imbalance of serotonin levels in the body affects the most basic functions in the body. Although, fruits and vegetables contain serotonin, to digest these foods you need a healthy digestive system. The digestive system follows its own schedule, controlled by the serotonin cycle.[27] The serotonin cycle, in turn, follows the circadian rhythm. This makes sunlight the most powerful and natural sustainer of life and health. Sunlight is pure medicine, and it's free.

Precautions:
Plan to avoid unnecessary or prolonged exposure to sunlight,

---

[27] See more details in "The Wonders Of Our Biological Rhythms," Chapter Five of *Timeless Secrets of Health and Rejuvenation*.

especially during the midday period in very hot climates, as well as protective clothing, sunglasses, and sunscreen. Many drugs, such as LIPITOR®/Atorvastatin, belladonna, furosemide, quinine, tetracycline, and doxycycline may make your eyes and skin sensitive to sunlight. Medication, stimulants such as caffeine, nicotine, and adrenaline, and recreational drugs can dilate the pupil, thereby allowing an excessive amount of light to enter the eye. This side effect may lead to the inappropriate use of sunglasses.

Highly acid-forming foods, including meat, eggs, cheese, fried foods, and sugar, may also make your eyes and skin prone to sun damage. Accordingly, you may find you can never leave the house without sunglasses. It is a pretty serious condition when the sun becomes so dangerous that you have to hide from it. The net result is, that not getting enough sunlight lowers your vitamin D and serotonin levels and thereby increases your risk of cancer and many other illnesses.

Also be aware that most cosmetics now contain UV-blocking chemicals. These include face creams, makeup products, moisturizers, lotions and anti-wrinkle creams.

If you feel you absolutely need a sunscreen product because you are unable to avoid the direct midday sun, make sure it has mostly natural ingredients in them, such as Aubrey Organics Active Full Spectrum Sunblock SPF 25. Still, it contains PABA Ester.

Other ingredients include: Titanium Dioxide, Coconut Fatty Acid Cream Base, Jojoba Butter, Organic Jojoba Oil, Organic Sunflower Oil, Organic Shea Butter, Organic Aloe Vera, White Camellia Oil, Lecithin, Canadian Willow herb Extract, Aubrey's Preservative (Citrus Seed Extract, Vitamins A, C and E), Silica, Jasmine Oil.

Coconut oil, shea butter or aloe vera may be sufficient for protection.

Pharmaceutical Drugs

Some of the most powerful direct and indirect causes of cancer are pharmaceutical drugs. Most drugs consist of a combination of synthetically derived chemicals that hook to the receptors of a cell in order to invoke or suppress specific responses that, for some reason, no longer occur naturally. Although this intervention on the cellular level sounds very logical and desirable, it can have serious consequences. It actually prevents your body from restoring its own natural responses when you try to determine the root causes of your health issues. After a while, your body will have no choice but to forsake the production of its own natural chemicals and become dependent on the drugs.

Take for an example, antidepressants. Many selective serotonin reuptake inhibitors (SSRIs) disturb the body's natural interactive cycles of serotonin/melatonin production, two of the body's most powerful brain hormones. As previously mentioned, serotonin is associated with positive moods, appetite, and satiety, and melatonin is, among other things, a sleep-inducer, providing the body with deep and rejuvenating sleep. By inhibiting the breakdown of serotonin in the body, these drugs disrupt the melatonin cycle and affect proper sleep induction. As the ongoing Nurses' Health Study[28] and other recent cancer research have shown, low melatonin levels in the blood greatly increase the risk of cancer. Melatonin controls a gene responsible for inducing normal cell death; low blood melatonin reduces that gene's activity, which in turn causes cells to live much longer than their normal lifespan. These uncontrolled cells become cancerous.

Antidepressants upset the most fundamental functions in the body, including the digestion of food and cell metabolism. Patients given the popular antidepressant *paraoxetine* (Paxil), for example, may suddenly feel much hungrier than usual and not feel full after eating. Thus, they eat more and more, a sure way to gain weight and become obese. Obesity is now considered the main risk factor for most chronic diseases, including heart

---

[28] The Nurses' Health Study, established in 1976 by Dr. Frank Speizer, and the Nurses' Health Study II, established in 1989 by Dr. Walter Willett, are the most definitive long-term epidemiological studies conducted to date on older women's health. The study has followed 121,700 female registered nurses since the mid-1970s to assess risk factors for cancer and cardiovascular disease (Wikipedia).

disease, cancer, and diabetes.

Some common antipsychotic drugs, such as *olanzapine* (Zyprexa), can bring about a weight gain of 30 pounds in a short period of time. These drugs boost *dopamine*, the hormone that causes food cravings. This class of drugs also decreases levels of *leptin*, a protein that suppresses appetite. In other words, those who take antidepressants may develop an unnaturally strong appetite that they cannot control by eating more. Think of the confusion and chaos this causes in the rest of the body, from producing more insulin and digestive juices, such as hydrochloric acid, bile, and enzymes, to having to eliminate ever-increasing amounts of harmful waste material. Elevated insulin secretions alone increase the risk of cancer in the body.

Other drugs, such as hormone replacement therapy (HRT) and the contraceptive pill or injections, lead to weight gain in up to 70% of users, once again interfering with the body's most basic functions. They also increase breast cancer risk. While this risk is considerably elevated during use of hormone medication, it drops back to the original level within about five years after a woman has stopped taking hormones. This is the result of a study by the German Cancer Research Center in Heidelberg and the University Hospitals of Hamburg-Eppendorf.

Bone-building drugs also cause weight gain. *Prednisone, cortisone,* and other steroids used to treat dozens of conditions, including asthma, lupus, and cancer, frequently cause weight gain because they increase appetite and force the body to retain fluids. Steroids cause just as many disorders as the conditions for which they are used, including liver cancer, heart disease, depression, hostility and aggression, eating disorders, stunted height, risk of HIV, acne, and dozens more.

Tamoxifen is a popular drug now used to prevent breast cancer recurrence in women. The drug can cause weight gain of up to 25 pounds, enough to dramatically increase the risk of other cancers, heart disease, and diabetes.

Many people, doctors and patients alike, perceive the ability of modern medicine to interfere with the body on the cellular level as a "medical miracle," but this miracle has brought more destruction into the world than it has prevented or eliminated. We have created an endless, vicious cycle by treating diseases that then cause other diseases, which, in turn, require further treatment. This self-perpetuating system of disease generation is largely due to the "medical miracle" that promises quick relief of symptoms at the expense of long-term suffering and ailments, and possibly, even death.

Although nearly one million people die each year from the side effects of medical treatments or medical errors, it is difficult for most people to forsake the illusion of a cure when learned scientists, doctors, pharmacists, the government, and drug makers so convincingly promise them a quick relief of their disease symptoms. It takes great courage, as well as trust in yourself, in your body's innate wisdom, and in nature, to heal what is only yours to heal. To heal cancer, the entire 'you' must become whole again, including your physical, mental, emotional, and spiritual self.

Beware of Popular Anticancer Drugs!

One of the most popular anticancer drugs is AVASTIN®, produced by the drug maker Genentech. In 2007, the drug sold a whopping $3.5 billion, with $2.3 billion in the United States. One course of treatment with Avastin can cost $100,000 per year. If a drug sells this well, it must be a very effective medicine, or so you could believe. However, when you read the following statement made by Genentech on their Avastin web site, www.avastin.com, you may wonder why it is prescribed at all: "Currently, no data are available that demonstrate an improvement in disease-related symptoms or increased survival with Avastin in breast cancer." The answer may lie in the fact that Avastin produces some of the worst side-effects a drug can produce, and that is good business. The thousands of doctors, hospital administrators, and health agencies that endorsed this killer drug either fell for the scam, or welcomed it.

Treatment with Avastin can result in the development of a potentially fatal Gastrointestinal (GI) perforation, a potentially fatal wound healing complication, a potentially fatal hemorrhage, fistula formation, strokes or heart problems (blood clots), hypertensive crisis (severe hypertension), reversible posterior leukoencephalopathy syndrome (nervous system and vision disturbances), neutropenia (a reduced white blood cell count that may increase the chance of infection), nephrotic syndrome (a sign of severe kidney malfunction), congestive heart failure, and many other bizarre symptoms or extreme illness.

Under great pressure, a recent FDA advisory panel has recommended that the drug Avastin should not be used to treat breast cancer, because it fails to provide enough benefit (which is none) to outweigh the risks. An FDA review of the drug concluded that Avastin did not significantly lengthen the lives of patients. On the contrary, it killed a number of patients.

An article published in the *New York Times* (July 5, 2008) raised some troubling questions about this drug. It says, "What does it mean to say the drug works? Is slowing the growth of tumors enough if life is not significantly prolonged or improved? How much evidence should there be before billions of dollars are spent on a drug? And when should cost be factored into the equation?" I will let a cancer patient answer that question:

In 2007, Jeanne Sather wrote on the web site, Assertivepatient.com, "Every three weeks, always on a Thursday afternoon, I amble on over to the cancer center for my IV treatment. (I also take Cytoxan, a chemo drug that comes in pill form, every day, plus a handful of other pills to help deal with the side effects and fringe benefits of being in cancer treatment – anxiety, high blood pressure, occasional depression, insomnia.) The total bill for each treatment session at the cancer center is something north of $20,000. The annual cost of my cancer care is more than $300,000. That's three hundred thousand dollars a year. Almost $30,000 a month to keep me alive....Both Herceptin and Avastin are made by Genentech Inc., a San Francisco Bay Area company that is doing very well, thank you. The reason they are so expensive is that they are new, and there are no generic versions available. So Genentech can charge whatever it wants, without competition, for these life-saving drugs....As a result of the high cost of Herceptin and Avastin, I am going to hit my lifetime max of $1 million on my health insurance before the end of 2007."

Beware of Arthritis Drugs!

Do Arthritis Drugs Cause Cancer? This is the title of an article published in the *New York Times*, June 5, 2008. As stated in the article, the FDA has received reports of 30 cases of cancer among children and young adults treated with drugs for rheumatoid arthritis, psoriasis, Crohn's disease, and other immune system diseases. The drugs involved are:

1. Enbrel, sold by Amgen and Wyeth
2. Remicade, sold by Johnson & Johnson and Schering-Plough
3. Humira, sold by Abbott Laboratories
4. Cimzia, sold by the Belgian company UCB

Because these drugs block part of the immune system, they naturally contribute to a higher risk of cancers and infections. The drugs' labels include a warning about a risk of lymphomas, which are cancers of immune system cells. The risk of develop-ing cancer as a result of taking arthritis medication is also prevalent among adults. One study found that those given Humira or Remicade to treat rheumatoid arthritis had 2.4 times the cancer rate of those in control groups. The most common cancers resulting from these drugs are lymphomas, skin, gastrointestinal, breast and lung cancers. Tuberculosis is listed as a side-effect, too. The question is whether it is better to live with psoriasis or arthritis, or to die from any of these other illnesses.

So who benefits from these drugs? You can draw your own conclusions. One year on Remicade costs about $12,000. The combined sales of Remicade, Humira and Enbrel in 2007 earned the drug makers $13 billion. You can easily heal the causes of arthritis, Crohn's disease, and psoriasis through cleansing of the liver, kidneys and colon, eliminating animal protein from the diet and eating a nutritious vegetarian diet, while adhering to a balanced lifestyle. I suffered from rheumatoid arthritis over 35 years ago, and once I knew what caused it, I healed it quickly without any medical aid. I appeal to all parents whose children are afflicted with arthritis, Crohn's disease, and similar disorders, to protect them against medical treatments designed to destroy their young and growing bodies. The "success" of these drugs is only measured by the degree of destruction or suppression of symptoms they can provide, but not by how much real healing they can induce.

Beware of Aspirin!

Who would have thought that the "harmless" aspirin pills millions of people swallow each day, every week, could actually cause one of the most serious cancers? A study at the Brigham and Women's Hospital (Boston, Massachusetts) of nearly 90,000 women, spanning 18 years of research, shows a 58% increased risk of pancreatic cancer when the participants took more than two aspirin a week. When the dosage exceeded 14 pills a week, the risk increased by 86%.

Avoid the Drug Trap!

It is becoming increasingly apparent that pharmaceutical drugs carry great risks. They kill at least 100,000 people in the U.S. each year. This figure could be much higher because only a fraction of drug-caused deaths are actually being reported by medical professionals. In nearly every case of death, the doctor issuing the death certificate writes down the name of the disease as the cause of death instead of the drug that was used to "treat" the disease. If doctors suddenly stopped prescribing drugs today, thousands of lives would be saved tomorrow. This truth has been known for many years.

In 1976, Los Angeles County registered a sudden reduction of its death rate by *18 percent* when many medical doctors went on strike against the increase of health insurance premiums for malpractice. In a study by Dr. Milton Roemer from the University of California, Los Angeles, 17 of the largest hospitals in the county showed a total of *60 percent* fewer operations during the period of the strike. When the doctors resumed work and medical activities went back to normal, death rates also returned to pre-strike levels.

A similar event took place in Israel in 1973. Doctors staged a one month strike and reduced their daily number of patients from 65,000 to 7,000. For the entire month, mortality rates in Israel were down 50 percent. This seems to happen whenever doctors go on strike. A two month work stoppage by doctors in the Columbian capital of Bogotá led to a 35 percent decline in deaths. This practically makes the medical profession, together with hospitals, the leading cause of death.

Besides killing patients, pharmaceutical drugs can cause permanent damage to the immune system, liver, kidneys, heart, brain and other organs. Taking prescription drugs can also send you to the emergency room. A Vancouver, Canada study has documented that 12% of emergency room (ER) visits were the direct result of problems with a pharmaceutical drug. In additon, the length of stay for those admitted to the hospital was significantly longer. The study, reported by the *Canadian Medical Association Journal*, was carried out at Vancouver General Hospital which has 995 beds and offers a wide range of services, including emergency care. The hospital treats 69,000 patients every year.

Pharmaceutical drugs are not designed to cure anything. They are designed to alleviate a symptom which is the body's way of dealing with an underlying physical/emotional imbalance that has not yet been resolved or dealt with. Basically, these drugs are designed to prevent your body from healing itself. The real problem is not that you have developed a symptom of an illness, but that you are being brainwashed to believe that the symptom is the problem, and that squashing it is all that you need in order to restore your health. The mindset that you have to pop a pill to fix a headache or heartburn because your doctor told you so is responsible for your reluctance to find out what causes these symptoms. Once the pain is gone, the problem is gone; at least this is what most people believe and what many doctors preach. The problem with this mindset is that it ignores the fact that these symptoms are warning signs that you are doing, being exposed to, eating, or neglecting something that coerces your body into a healing response (symptom).

A symptom of pain or discomfort is not an illness in itself to be "cured" by a pill, wrongly called "medicine." Real medicine supports and encourages the body to complete the healing process it has already begun (as indicated by the symptom). Pharmaceutical drugs are made to suppress the body's ability to heal, which reduces or eliminates the symptoms but also fortifies the origins of the illness. This makes regular symptom-squashing (medical treatment) a leading cause of disease, including cancer. I recommend that you don't enter the drug trap; it only pushes you into a vicious cycle from which it is difficult to escape.

Chapter Three

Demystifying Cancer

Connecting the Pieces

Mary visited me when she was 39 years old. One year earlier she had been diagnosed with advanced breast cancer. Her oncologist had prescribed the standard routine treatments for cancer—radiation and chemotherapy—but to no avail. Shortly afterward, he advised her to undergo a mastectomy of her right breast. The operation took place shortly before her menstrual period began. Much to her relief, her doctors informed her that they "got all the cancer" and the situation was now under control. Little did her doctors know that, according to the science of *chronobiology,*[29] the risk of the cancer recurring is four times higher in women who undergo surgery one week before or during menstruation than for those who have surgery at other points in their cycle. While menstruating, a woman's immunity and iron levels are measurably lower. Her body is, therefore, not able to destroy all the cancer cells left over from surgery. Hence, the woman is at high risk for cancer cells developing in other parts of her body.

Not surprisingly, one year after her mastectomy, Mary began to complain of severe pain in her lower spine and left knee. Ten years earlier she had been diagnosed with *cervical spondylosis*[30] in her lower spine, caused by abnormal outgrowth and ossified

---

[29] Chronobiology is the science of "body clocks" attuned to the earth's cycles and encoded in our cells. The human body is endowed with at least 100 such "clocks," which are unrelated to our watch time. The circadian rhythm, for example, is responsible for numerous hormonal cycles that determine our hunger, moods, metabolism, and rate of growth and aging. For more information, see *Timeless Secrets of Health and Rejuvenation.*

[30] Spondylosis is spinal degeneration and deformity of the joint(s) of two or more vertebrae.

cartilage around the margins of the joints of the vertebral column. This time, however, an examination revealed that she had developed bone cancer in her lower spine and left knee. The breast surgery and resulting suppression of the immune system had, as so often is the case, encouraged millions of cancer cells to develop in other already weakened parts of Mary's body. Therefore, cancer cells began to grow in her lower spine where the resistance to cancer formation was particularly low.

Mary had also been suffering from severe menstrual problems for as long as she remembered. In addition, she had been diagnosed with anemia. However, despite taking iron tablets regularly for years, which caused her frequent nausea and stomach cramps, she remained anemic. She told me that her digestive system had "never worked properly," and constipation often lasted for as many as three to five days in a row. My examination revealed that her liver was filled with thousands of intrahepatic stones.

Mary also mentioned that she had received multiple antibiotic treatments over the years for all kinds of infections. It is a well-established fact that regular use of antibiotics sharply increases breast cancer risk. According to cancer research, the risk of breast cancer is twice as high among women who have taken 25 or more rounds of antibiotics of any variety over a 17-year period, in comparison with women who have used no antibiotics at all.

Mary was brought up with a lot of candy, cake, ice cream and chocolate. A number of recent studies have linked a greater risk of breast cancer among women to a diet high in sugar (especially soft drinks and popular sweet desserts). Scientists now believe that the extra insulin released to process the simple starches and sugars found in these foods causes cells to divide and estrogens in the blood to rise. Both of these factors (cellular division and blood estrogens) can contribute to cancer growth.

Cancer's Emotional Causes

Mary experienced a very sad childhood because her parents had great problems relating to one another. When I asked her, she could not remember even a single instance when there had not been tension between her parents. Being a very sensitive person at heart, she took everything more seriously than her more extroverted brother did, and consequently felt insecure, frightened, and depressed. With a painful smile on her face, Mary said that she had always felt torn between her mother and father, and could not choose which one to favor.

Eating meals with her parents was particularly difficult. She was forced to sit and eat with them while being tormented by a very tense atmosphere. Sometimes everyone would keep quiet, in an attempt not to arouse any new conflicts. Today she has a strong aversion to, and fear of, food and she gobbles it down very quickly, often while standing or driving.

Mary also faces great difficulties at work. In her job as a teacher, she feels that her students are allowed to take their frustrations out on her, but she has to keep hers all inside. When she returns home, though, she shouts at her own children, which creates much guilt in her. She wants to be a good mother but believes she is not; she just doesn't know how to be kind to her children. Mary also told me that she never really wanted to be a classroom teacher; she always dreamed of becoming a gymnastics coach.

The frustration of not fulfilling her desires was a major cause of Mary's cancer. Right from the beginning of her life she was taught to conform to the social system, which for her meant that she always had to do what she was told. Deep inside herself she had dreams that she could never fulfill because she did not want to stir up tension or make other people think badly of her.

In order to keep the peace, Mary went along with what her parents demanded of her, but inside she was boiling with rage. When Mary walked into my office that morning, she gave me a beautiful smile which did not reveal the pain she was feeling inside. She had learned to conceal her inner world from the outer world. It was not so much the physical pain in her body that hurt her; it was all the bottled-up frustration, fear, and insecurity that threatened the sensitive feelings of love and peace in her heart. The physical pain merely reminded her of the profound emotional heartache from which she had been suffering for so long.

113

Her endless attempts to suppress or hide her true inner feelings through both childhood and adulthood shaped a personality that eventually required a disease to bring it all to some kind of conclusion.

Torn between her parents for many years and trying to please both of them, Mary had never been bold enough to make a choice that would please herself and herself only. The division within her heart sapped all her energy and happiness. The cancer started in her divided heart, in all the unexpressed grief and frustration that had filled her early life.

It's All Psychosomatic

Whatever happens in our emotional body also occurs in our physical body. The real cancer is a trapped and isolated emotion, a feeling of "having no choice." Through the mind/body connection, any repressed feelings of wanting and deserving harmony, peace, stability, and a simple sense of joy in life are translated into appropriate biochemical responses in the body. This effectively deprives the body cells of all these positive qualities as well. Cells are not physical machines that have no feelings, no sense of "I"-ness, no reaction to external changes or threats. The emotional suffocation caused so much anger and frustration in Mary, that for fear of not being loved or liked by others, including her parents, she targeted these negative emotions at her own body. Her "toxic" mind translated into a toxic body, and it threatened Mary's very survival. She threatened the health of the cells of her body by keeping her most important thoughts and feelings to herself.

Whatever you keep to yourself out of fear of being criticized or hurt, actually turns into poisons in the body. These poisons are so strong that if you cried and put your tears on a snake's skin, they would burn holes into it. [I have actually seen this phenomenon demonstrated when I lived in Africa.] Tears of joy, on the other hand, do not have any poison in them.

The constant tension, which Mary experienced during dinnertime at her parental home, had greatly impaired her digestive functions. Under stress or tension, the blood vessels supplying the organs of the digestive system become tight and restricted, preventing them from digesting even the healthiest of foods. Furthermore, to eat while you are emotionally upset suppresses the secretion of balanced amounts of digestive juices. Whenever you feel angry or upset, your bile flora (beneficial bacteria that keep bile balanced) are altered, which predisposes bile to coagulate. Constant emotional strain leads to stone formation in the bile ducts of the liver and in the gallbladder. The resulting curbed secretion of bile lowers *Agni*, the digestive fire. Mary still associates the eating of her meals with the tension she experienced while sitting at the parental dinner table. Her unconscious attempt to avoid everything that has to do with food and eating, programs her body to do the same. The body cannot properly digest and absorb foods that are eaten in a hurry, hence the accumulation of large quantities of toxic waste in her small and large intestines. Chronic constipation and the poor absorption of nutrients, including fats, calcium, zinc, magnesium, and vitamins had increasingly depleted and weakened her bone tissue, bone marrow, and reproductive functions.

When the reproductive tissue, which maintains the genetic blueprint (DNA) of the cells, is starved of oxygen and nutrients, it is only a matter of time before normal and healthy cells begin to mutate their genes and divide abnormally in order to survive the "famine." Normally, a host of immune cells, pancreatic enzymes, and vitamins break down cancer cells in the body, wherever they appear. However, most of the digestive enzymes are "used up" quickly when the diet is rich in animal protein, such as beef, pork, poultry, fish, eggs, cheese, and milk, as well as sugar-enriched foods. Mary practically lived on these foods. Having suffered from poor digestion and constipation for most of her life, Mary's body was practically deprived of all of these natural antidotes to cancer cells. Cancers are much more likely to occur among those whose digestive functions are continually disturbed and who are deprived of a sense of emotional wellbeing than in those whose digestive system is efficient and who generally have a happy disposition.

The spondylosis of Mary's lower spine signifies the weakening of her internal and external support system; it manifested in direct response to the lack of support and encouragement by her parents. Mary's body slumps forward while she sits and looks half its size. She looks like a scared child, without confidence and trust. Her posture suggests that she is trying to protect her heart from being hurt again. In addition, her breathing is shallow and insufficient, as if she does not want to be noticed and possibly criticized or disapproved of by her parents. The knees serve as a support system for the entire body. A lifetime of "giving in" and "not standing up for herself and her desires" manifested as the knee problems she developed over the years.

Mary's Successful Remedies

Japanese research has shown that cancer patients whose cancerous tumors went into spontaneous remission, often within less than 24 hours, experienced a profound transformation in their attitude toward themselves before the sudden cure occurred. Mary needed to make several major changes in her life, one of which was to find a new job, even if this meant taking a pay cut. While Mary was still highly susceptible to stressful situations and chaotic noise, the tense atmosphere present at her school was hardly conducive to the healing process. She also needed to spend more time in nature, walk in the sun and on the beach, paint her impressions, listen to her favorite music, and devote some time to quietness and meditation every day.

In addition to following an Ayurvedic daily routine and diet, Mary began to use a number of cleansing procedures to rid her colon of stagnant, old fecal matter and to purify the blood, liver, and connective tissue from accumulated toxins. The liver flush produced thousands of stones that had affected both her liver and gallbladder for at least 15 - 20 years.

The most important thing for Mary was to become more conscious about everything in her life. This included eating, emotional releases, and listening to her body's signals for thirst, hunger, and tiredness. She needed to become aware of her needs and desires and begin to fulfill them whenever possible. The most important realization she had to make was that she did not need to do anything that did not please her. Giving herself permission to make mistakes, and not judge herself if she made them, was essential therapy for her.

Mary's friends and family also needed to understand that she was at a very crucial stage of recovery where every positive thought and feeling toward her could serve as a tremendous support system, one that she had never experienced when she was young. Mary started to improve steadily six months after she adopted about 60% percent of my recommended advice. Today she feels that the disease has brought her a deeper understanding of life and has led to an inner awakening she had never experienced before. Today, while free of cancer, Mary continues to improve and grow in confidence and self-acceptance.

Cancer—A Response to Rejection

Jeromy has *Hodgkin's* disease, which is the most common *lymphoma*. Lymphomas are malignant neoplasms of lymphoid tissue that vary in growth rate, also known as lymph cancer. Contemporary medicine cannot explain what causes the disease. Hodgkin's disease usually begins in adolescence or between 50 and 70 years of age.

When Jeromy was 22 years old, he noticed two enlarged lymph nodes in his neck. A few days later, he was diagnosed with Hodgkin's disease. In some people, the disease leads to death within a few months, but others have few signs of it for many years. Jeromy was one of them. Being a Kapha type[31], he has a very athletic and strong body and is naturally endowed with a lot of stamina and physical endurance. His naturally slow metabolic rate can be considered responsible for the slow advancement of the illness.

Jeromy received his first chemotherapy treatment in 1979, soon after he was diagnosed with lymphoma, but there was no

---

[31] See details about the Ayurvedic body types, Vata, Pitta and Kapha, in *Timeless Secrets of Health and Rejuvenation*. The Kapha type has the strongest bones and muscles of the three types.

detectable improvement in his condition. In 1982, his doctors added multiple radiation treatments to the regular chemotherapy, but these produced severe side effects, including the loss of all body hair and Jeromy's sense of taste. His distress was considerable. Yet, despite numerous traumatic experiences caused by the various treatments during the following 14 years, Jeromy was not willing to give into depression and desperation. His strong fighting spirit permitted him to continue his work as a general manager of a successful business enterprise.

Through the Ayurvedic Pulse Reading method and Eye Interpretation (iridology)[32], I was able to determine that from a very early age, Jeromy's digestive functions and lymph drainage had begun to decline rapidly. His liver showed the presence of a large number of intrahepatic stones. As it turned out, Jeromy had gone through a very traumatic experience when he was four years old, although at first he had difficulty remembering it. According to Jeromy, the most emotionally stressful event for him occurred at age 21, when his long-term girlfriend suddenly left him for another man. Exactly one year before she left, he discovered the lymph swellings in his neck. The rejection by his girlfriend was one of the most heart-breaking experiences of his life. Yet this experience merely triggered the memory of an even more painful rejection.

Fighting the Ghost of Memory

Jeromy was born in a developing country with an unstable political situation. When he reached the age of four, his parents sent him to a boarding school in another developing country, for his own safety. Unable to understand the reasons behind this move, he felt that his parents had stopped loving him and no longer wanted him around. All he remembered was the feeling of being cut off from what he considered his lifeline—the closeness with his parents. Although his parents believed that sending him away was in Jeromy's best interest, he suddenly lost the love of

---

[32] Diagnostic methods used to determine any existing imbalances in the body and mind.

the most important people in his life, at an age when he needed it most. His little world had collapsed on this first "black" day in his life, and his body's main functions subsequently began to decline.

Jeromy spent much of his life trying to prove to his parents that he was worthy of their love. He was not aware, however, of his incessant drive to succeed in life. He proudly told me that he never gave up in life and that he refused to allow anything to get him down. One part of him never acknowledged that he was gravely ill. His physical appearance, except for being bald, did not reveal the battle his body was fighting. He invested all of his energy and time in his work, and he was very good at it.

To heal himself physically, though, Jeromy needed to become aware of the "rejected child" within him. He had buried that part of himself in the most hidden depths of his subconscious when he was four years old, and a second time, when he was 21 years old and his girlfriend left him. This second rejection amplified the already deep hurt caused by what he considered a rejection by his parents.

The body stores all the experiences we have in some kind of invisible "filing cabinets." Accordingly, all the feelings of anger we have in life go into one file, sad events are placed into another, and rejections are deposited in yet a different file. These impressions are not recorded and stored according to linear time, but are compiled in terms of similarity. They feed "the ghost of memory" and give it more and more energy. Once a file is "filled up," even a small event can trigger a devastating eruption and awaken the ghost of memory, thereby giving it a life of its own. This had happened in Jeromy's life.

The abandonment that Jeromy had experienced as a four year old reawakened in his awareness when his girlfriend left him. By ignoring or denying the fact that this rejection had ever taken place, he unconsciously directed his body to create the identical response, which was a cancer in the very system that is responsible for neutralizing and removing harmful waste in the body – the lymphatic system. Unable to get rid of the ghost of memory, which consisted of deep-seated fear and anger from feeling abandoned, Jeromy was also no longer able to free himself of dead, turned-over cells and metabolic waste products.[33] Both his liver and gallbladder had accumulated thousands of gallstones, which nearly suffocated him. His body had no choice but to give physical expression to the cancer that had tortured Jeromy's heart and mind for so many years.

Letting Go of the Need to Fight

All events in life that appear to be negative are, in fact, unique opportunities to become more complete and whole inside and to move forward in life. Whenever we need to give ourselves more love, time, and appreciation but fail to fulfil these essential needs, someone or something in our life will push us in that direction. Feeling rejected by or being disappointed and angry with another person, highlights a lack in taking responsibility for the negative things that happen to us. Blaming oneself or someone else for an unfortunate situation results in the feeling of being a victim and is likely to manifest itself as disease. Moreover, if we cannot understand the accompanying message of our illness, we may even have to face death to appreciate life or living.

Cancer, in an unconventional sense, is a way out of a dead-locked situation that paralyzes the heart of a person. It helps to break down old, rigid patterns of guilt and shame that keep a person imprisoned and bound by a constant sense of low self-worth. The current medical approach does not target this major issue behind cancer, but the "disease process" does, provided it is allowed to take its course. Chemotherapy, radiation, and surgery encourage a victim mentality in the patient and are unlikely to heal the root causes of this affliction. Miracle cures happen when the patient frees himself or herself of the need for victim-hood and self-attack. When the person's inner sense of wellbeing and self-acceptance are strong, external problems fail to have a major disruptive impact. Thus, removing the external problems in life alone may not be sufficient to induce a spontaneous remission; an

---

[33] To be healthy, the human body has to remove over 30 billion dead, worn-out cells and a large amount of metabolic waste every day.

accompanying inward change is also essential.

Jeromy needed to give himself the love and appreciation he did not feel he was getting from his parents. He also needed to make room for enjoyment and pleasure, taking time for himself, for meditation, for self-reflection, for being in nature and sensing the joy and energy it is able to evoke in us. Cancer cells are cells fighting to survive in a "hostile," toxic environment. Letting go of the need to fight in life reprograms the DNA of the body, changing its course of warfare and eventual annihilation to one of healthy reproduction. Not needing to fight for their survival gives the cancer cells a chance to be accepted again by the entire "family" of cells in the body. Cancer cells are normal cells that have been rejected by what they consider home. They are deprived of proper nourishment and support. In their desperation to survive, they grab anything they can find to live on, even cellular waste products and toxins. This practically turns them into "outcasts."

However, just as *we* want to be loved, cancer cells also need to know that they are loved. Cutting them out of the body through surgery, or destroying them with poisonous drugs or deadly radiation, adds even more violence to the body than it already has to deal with. To live in health and peace, we especially need to be friends with the cells of our body, including cancer cells. The saying, "Love thy enemy," applies to cancer cells just as it applies to people. The cause of Jeromy's cancer was a lack of self-appreciation, a feeling of not being loved and wanted, of not feeling worthy or good enough. By waiting for his parents to show him their love, he effectively denied this love to himself. Jeromy came to realize that his disease was, in fact, a great blessing in disguise that could help him find and love himself for the very first time.

If we could only see that what we call disease is a perfect representation of our inner world, we would pay more attention to what is going on inside rather than trying to fix something that does not really need fixing. Cancer, as hard as this may be to understand, has profound meaning to it. Its purpose is not to destroy but to heal what is no longer whole.

Cancer—A Powerful Healer

A few years ago, a woman posted a message on my Cure-zone.com forum *Ask Andreas Moritz*[34] inquiring how she could support her twin sister who had just been diagnosed with cancer. She mentioned that her sister had rejected her almost her entire life. She also told me that she was trying her best to be strong for her sister. I replied that being strong was not actually what her sister and she needed at this time. This is what I wrote to her: "Cancer is most often caused by trying to be strong outwardly while not expressing or acknowledging the weakness and vulnerability that one feels inside. What your sister needs most from you now is to provide her with a mirror of herself. Show her how you really feel inside. Show her your own guilt, your poor self-worth, and your tears of constant rejection, so that she can start seeing these in herself and developing the courage to release the trapped emotions she has locked up inside her body. If you wish her to heal from this, show her all your weaknesses, and allow yourself to cry for her and for yourself. It will motivate her to do the same."

I continued explaining that her sister's cancer was merely an unconscious attempt to keep everything trapped inside, including foods, waste matter, resentment, anger, fear, and other negative feelings and emotions. "For this reason," I wrote, "to heal cancer, one must turn inside out and let the world see what one is hiding from (due to a false sense of shame and guilt). Guilt is a completely unjustified and unnecessary emotion because human beings are actually incapable of wrongdoing, although this is nearly impossible to understand when one does not recognize the larger picture of all things[35]. You can actually never cause someone else's problems unless the affected other person is

---

[34] The forum is called *Ask Andreas Moritz* and is found on the health website *Curezone.com*. If offers Andreas's answers to thousands of questions (search archives).

[35] See the author's book *Lifting the Veil of Duality—Your Guide to Living Without Judgment* to understand how "mistakes" and "wrongdoing" are learned negative concepts and beliefs surrounding experiences that could be immensely beneficial in our lives.

allowing or requesting it (unconsciously) by direct decree of their Higher Self[36]. The guilt (of not loving or caring about her own twin sister) consists of powerful negative energies that started congesting and attacking the cells of her own body. The cancer is her chosen alternative way to break down the guilt in her heart—a way for her to bring to her conscious attention the false subconscious beliefs of past wrongdoing."

During conversations with cancer patients, I often raise the subject of death, which inevitably is something they face. I suggest to them that they cannot really die; nobody can. Physical death is only a tangible, real experience for those who are left behind. It is a non-reality for the self of the person whose body passes away. Physical death does nothing to the conscious being that resides in, and expresses itself, through the physical body. A snake that glides out of its old skin is not concerned about a part of its body dying and falling off. As long as our sense of "I" remains, which it always will, physical death cannot destroy us. In fact, death is a non-experience, and therefore, an illusion that is real only for those who rely on their physical senses to determine what they believe. When a loved one suddenly disappears from our lives as a result of physical death, we naturally grieve for him or her, are sad, or feel empty inside. Whereas the grief and sadness are real, the reason for these emotions is not. The vanishing of someone occurs only relative to the observer, but nothing happens at all to the person who "disappears;" he remains who he has always been, just not in a physical body.

I have personally died several times (had near death experiences)[37] during bouts of severe illness or trauma. My father had

---

[36] Each person has a Higher Self guiding one's physical existence down to the minutest detail.

[37] During one episode of malaria in India, my soul or consciousness departed/detached from my physical body and "rose," while I was completely aware of what was happening. I experienced no fear of dying and sensed no loss of any kind. I was in a state of incredible clarity that I could know anything if I wanted to. A doctor confirmed that my heart had stopped. I had a similar experience during a fainting spell. My heart stopped for five minutes before I returned to my physical body.

the same experience, but neither of us had the sensation of dying. In reality, quite the contrary occurred: the intensity of being alive, awake, and conscious of everything became so much more heightened, that the sense of dying was as remote as the faraway galaxies. By contrast, being pulled back into the sick physical body was rather like dying. When I buried my mother, it was a day of celebration, just the way she wanted it. Instead of feeling sorry for ourselves, we can actually honor the departed soul by being happy for them. The only pain and regret you feel when you die physically is that the loved ones left behind don't share in your incredible joy and expansiveness of being truly free and alive.

Nothing in the self or of the self goes anywhere when someone goes through a death experience. "Accordingly," I wrote to this woman, "more important than continuing to live in her physical body is whether she manages to make peace with herself, because she will carry everything with her, except the flesh of the physical body. Whether she is ready to accept and embrace herself as she is, and thereby heal herself from the unconscious act of self-destruction, is completely up to her, and nobody can or should make that decision for her. As hard as it may be to understand, she is responsible for everything that is happening to her. The only thing you can do for her is to show her who *you* are and how *you* feel. This could be just the catalyst she needs in order to go through her own transformation. Telling her what to do is most certainly not what she needs. By forgiving and, thus, healing yourself, you can be the best help to her, provided she has it in her to be open and ready to heal herself."

If you have a loved one who has cancer, you can play a very important role in his or her healing process. By opening up your own heart to him and sharing your own fears and perceived weaknesses, you are encouraging him to open up his heart to you as well. Allow the person to shed as many tears as he needs to, and do not try to pacify him and tell him, "It is all going to be okay." Let him have his experience of pain, despair, confusion, loneliness, hopelessness, anger, fear, guilt, or shame. Cancer does not actually generate these emotions, but it may bring them from the subconscious to more conscious levels of feeling and understanding. If the afflicted person knows that he or she can have all these feelings without having to hide them from you or push them right back inside, cancer can become a very powerful means of self-healing. Just staying by your friend's side without judging or trying to take away his pain will make you a better healer than any doctor could possibly be.

The Power of Resolving Conflict Situations

Unresolved conflict is most likely the starting point of any illness, including cancer. The body always uses the stress response to cope with the traumatizing effect of conflict. According to a study released by the *Journal of Biological Chemistry* on March 12, 2007, the stress hormone *epinephrine* changes prostate and breast cancer cells in ways that may make them resistant to cell death. The researchers found that epinephrine levels increase sharply in response to stressful situations and can remain continuously elevated during long periods of stress or depression. They discovered that when cancer cells are exposed to epinephrine, a protein called BAD, which causes cell death, becomes inactive. This means that emotional stress may not only trigger or contribute to the development of cancer, but also undermine or reduce the effectiveness of cancer treatments.

The German university professor, Ryke Geerd Hamer, M.D., discovered during routine CT scans of over 20,000 cancer patients, that each of them had a lesion in a certain part of the brain that looked like concentric rings on a shooting target or like the surface of water after a stone has been dropped into it. This distortion in the brain is known as "HAMER herd." Dr. Hamer, now living in Spain, found that these lesions resulted from a serious, acute-dramatic and isolating conflict-shock-experience in the patient. Whenever the conflict was resolved, the CT image changed; an edema developed, and finally scar tissue formed. Naturally, the cancers would stop growing, become inactive, and disappear.

Simply by helping patients to resolve their acute conflicts and supporting the body during this healing phase, Dr. Hamer achieved an exceptionally high success rate with his cancer therapy. According to public record, after 4 to 5 years of receiving his simple treatment, 6,000 out of 6,500 patients with mostly advanced cancer were still alive.

Cancer is "Not Loving Yourself"

Many cancer patients have devoted their entire lives to helping and supporting others. Their selfless service can be a very noble quality, depending upon the motivation behind it. If they sacrifice and neglect their own wellbeing to avoid facing any shame, guilt, or unworthiness within themselves, they are actually cutting off the very limb they are hanging on to. They are "selflessly" devoted to please others so that, in return, they may be loved and appreciated for their contributions. This, however, serves as an unconscious acknowledgment of *not loving oneself.* This may lock up unresolved issues, fears, and feelings of unworthiness in the cellular memory of the organs and tissues in the body.

"Love thy neighbor as thou lovest thyself" is one of the most basic requirements for curing cancer. This phrase means that we can only love others as much as we are able to love and appreciate ourselves, no less and no more. To be able to truly love someone without cords of attachment and possessiveness, one has to fully accept oneself with all the flaws, mistakes and inadequacies one may have. The degree to which we are able to care about the wellbeing of our body, mind, and spirit determines the degree to which we are able to care about other people, too. By being critical of ourselves, or disliking the way we look, behave, or feel, we close down our heart and feel unworthy and ashamed. To avoid exposing our shadow self (the part of our self we do not like) to others out of fear of rejection, we try to win over the love of others by pleasing them. This way, we assume, we can receive the love we are unable to give to ourselves. However, this approach fails to work in the long term.

Your body always follows the commands given by your mind. Such inner promptings as your thoughts, emotions, feelings, desires, beliefs, drives, likes, and dislikes serve as the software with which your cells are programmed on a daily basis. Through the mind/body connection, your cells have no choice but to obey the orders they receive via your subconscious or conscious mind. As DNA research has recently proved, you can literally alter your DNA's genetic setting and behavior within a matter of a moment. Your DNA listens to every word you utter to yourself, and it feels every emotion you experience. Moreover, it responds to all of them. You program yourself every second of the day, consciously and unconsciously. If you choose to, you can rewrite the program in any way you want to, provided you are truly self-aware. Once you know who you truly are, you cannot help but love, accept and honor yourself. You can no longer judge yourself for making mistakes in life, for not being perfect, for not always being how others want you to be. Seeing yourself in this light, you send a signal of love to your cells. The bonding effect of love unites differences and keeps everything together in harmony, including the cells of your body. When love, which should not be confused with neediness or attachment, is no longer a daily-experienced reality, the body begins to disintegrate and become sick.

The increase of love is the main purpose of our existence here on Earth. Those who love themselves are also able to love others, and vice versa. They thrive on sharing their full heart with other people, animals, and the natural environment. People who accept themselves fully have no real fear of death; when their time comes to die, they leave peacefully without any regrets or remorse in their hearts.

Whenever we close our hearts to ourselves, we become lonely, and the body begins to become weak and diseased. It is known that widows and people who are socially isolated, or who have nobody with whom to share their deepest feelings, are the most prone to developing cancer.

Your body cells are the most intimate "neighbors" you can have, and they need to feel your love and self-acceptance, to know that they are a part of you and that you care about them. Giving yourself an oil massage, going to sleep on time, eating nutritious foods, and engaging in other healthy daily routines are simple, but powerful messages of love that motivate your cells to function in harmony with each other. They are also messages that keep the elimination of toxins flawless and efficient. There is nothing unscientific about this. You can visit a number of hospitals and ask the patients whether they felt good about their life prior to falling ill. The overwhelming response would be, "No." Without being a medical researcher, you would have conducted one of the most important research studies anyone could ever do. You would have stumbled over the most common cause of ill health which is, "not loving yourself," or, to use a different expression, "not being happy about how your life turned out." Not being happy or satisfied in life is perhaps the most severe form of emotional stress to which you could possibly subject yourself. It is, in fact, a major risk factor for many diseases, including cancer.

A recently published study suggests that severe emotional stress can triple the risk of breast cancer. One hundred women who had a breast lump were interviewed before they knew that they had breast cancer. One in two who had the illness had suffered a major traumatic life event, such as bereavement, within the previous five years. The effects of emotional stress or unhappiness can severely impair digestion, elimination, and immunity, thus leading to a dangerously high level of toxicity in the body. Just ridding the body of cancer through "weapons of mass destruction" fails to remove the unresolved emotional pain behind it.

Chapter Four

Body Intelligence in Action

Cancer Cannot Kill You

Cancer, like any other disease, is not a clearly definable phe-nomenon that suddenly and randomly appears in some part or parts of the body like mushrooms popping out of the ground. Cancer is rather the result of many crises of toxicity that have, as their common origin, one or more energy-depleting influences. Stimulants, emotional trauma, repressed emotions, an irregular lifestyle, dehydration, nutritional deficiencies, overeating, stress reactions, a lack of deep sleep, the accumulation of heavy metals (especially from amalgam tooth fillings), exposure to chemicals, and a lack of sunshine are among the factors that hinder the body in its effort to remove metabolic waste, toxins, and 30 billion turned-over cells each day. When these dead cells accumulate in any part of the body, this naturally leads to a number of progres-sive responses that include irritation, swelling, hardening, inflammation, ulceration, and abnormal cell growth. Like every other disease, cancer is but a toxicity crisis. It marks the body's final attempt to rid itself of septic poisons and acidic compounds that have accumulated because the body was not able to properly remove metabolic waste, toxins, and decomposing cells.

Cancer always manifests as the result of an already toxic state in the body. It is never the cause of a disease, but rather a reaction to a far-advanced, unhealthful physical condition. Treating cancer as if it were the cause of a disease is like cleaning a dirty pot [the toxin-infested body] with filthy mud [the slew of poisons contained in the chemotherapy cocktail]. Obviously, using toxic substances to treat a body that is already struggling to survive due to an overload of toxins will never bring about the desired result of a clean, well-functioning body. Of course, you can throw away the pot and thereby solve the problem, but when it comes to preparing a new meal, you will face an even bigger problem: you have nothing to cook your food in. Similarly, by killing the cancer we almost always kill the patient, too; perhaps not right away, but gradually.

Despite huge efforts and expenditures by the medical establishment (for whatever reasons), mortality rates from cancer have not decreased in over 50 years. Although surgery can certainly help neutralize or eliminate a lot of the septic poison kept in check by a tumor mass and in a good number of cases improve the condition, neither surgery nor the other two main treatment procedures (chemotherapy and radiation) remove the cause(s) of cancer. What happened to Tony Snow can happen to anyone. A cancer patient may return home after a "successful" treatment, relieved and obviously "cured," but continue to deplete his body's energy and to gather toxins as he did before (by eating the same harmful foods and living the same taxing lifestyle). The immune system, already battered by one traumatic intervention, may not make it through a second one. However, if the patient dies, it is not actually the cancer that has killed him, but rather its untreated cause(s). Given the current extremely small remission rate for most medically treated cancers (7%), the promises made to cancer patients that by destroying their tumors they will also be cured are deceptive, to say the least. Patients are rarely being told what turns a normal, robust cell into a weak, damaged, abnormal cell.

Tumor cells are cells that "panic" due to a lack of food, water, oxygen, and space. Survival is their basic genetic instinct, just as it is ours. To survive in such an acidic, unsupportive environment, the defective cells are forced to mutate and begin devouring everything they can get hold of to sustain themselves, including toxins. They leach more nutrients, such as glucose, magnesium, and calcium from the tissue fluid than they would need to if they were normally growing cells. To produce the same amount of energy as a healthy cell makes, a cancer cell requires 15 times the amount of glucose. Cancer cells need to ferment glucose, which is a very inefficient and wasteful method of producing cellular energy, similar to the burning of fossil fuels on this planet. Their healthier neighboring cells, however, begin to waste away gradually in the process, and eventually an entire organ becomes dysfunctional due to exhaustion, malnutrition, or wasting. Cancerous tumors always look for more energy to divide and multiply cells. Sugar is one of their favorite energy-supplying foods. Craving sugar can indicate excessive cell activity, and many people who eat lots of sugar end up growing tumors in their body.

It seems obvious that cancer cells must be responsible for the death of a person; this is the main reason that almost the entire medical approach is geared toward destroying them. However, cancer cells are far from being the culprits, just as blocked arteries are not the real reason for heart disease. In fact, cancer cells help a highly congested body survive a little longer than it would without them. What possible reason could the immune system have to ignore cancer cells that cluster together to form a tumor mass—cells that it could easily destroy? The only reasonable explanation is that these cells are doing a critical job in a body filled with toxic waste. Nature provides a clear example of this when one considers the function of poisonous mushrooms. A mushroom is the fleshy, spore-bearing fruiting body of a fungus. Would you call such a poisonous mushroom "vicious" or "evil" just because it could kill you if you ate it? No, in fact, those mushrooms in the forest attract and absorb poisons from the soil, water, and air. They form an essential part of the ecological system in our natural world. Although the cleansing effect produced by these mushrooms is hardly noticeable, it allows for the healthy growth of the forest and its natural inhabitants. In fact, the survival of the entire planet depends on the existence of mushrooms. Likewise, cancer cells are not at all vicious; in fact, they serve a similarly good purpose of absorbing some of the toxins in the body that would otherwise kill the person immediately. It is never the primary choice of normal, healthy cells to suddenly become "poisonous" or malignant, but it is the next best choice they have to avoid an immediate catastrophe in the body. If the body dies, it is not because of cancer, but because of the underlying reasons that led up to it.

To continue to do their increasingly difficult job, these tumor cells need to grow, even if it is at the expense of other healthy cells. Without their activity, an organ may suddenly lose its already weakened structure and collapse. Some of the cancer cells may even leave a tumor site and enter the lymph fluid, which carries them to other parts of the body that also suffer an equally high degree of toxicity or acidosis. The spreading of cancer cells is known as *metastasis*. However, cancer cells are programmed to settle only in the "fertile" ground of high toxicity (acidity), a milieu in which they can survive and continue their unusual rescue mission. They have mutated to be able to live in a toxic, non-oxygenated environment where they help to neutralize at least some of the trapped metabolic waste, such as lactic acid and decomposing cellular debris. Given these circumstances, it would be a fatal mistake by the immune system to destroy these "estranged" cells that are doing a vital part of the immune system's work. Without the tumor's presence, large amounts of septic poison, resulting from the accumulated corpses of decomposing cells, would perforate the capillary walls, seep into the blood, and kill the person within a matter of hours or days. It is important to remember that cancer cells are still the body's cells. If they were no longer needed, one simple command from the DNA would stop them from dividing wildly.

Tumors cannot kill anyone (unless they obstruct a vital pathway). We have already established that cancer cells contain no weapons to destroy anything. In additon, the vast majority of cells in a tumor are not cancerous at all. Cancer cells are unable to form tissues; only healthy cells can. A tumor could not exist without normal cells holding it together. If accounted for, the number of cancer cells contained in a prostate or lung tumor, for example, would be too insignificant to endanger the life of a person.

Tumors act like sponges for the poisons that circulate and accumulate in the blood, lymph and tissue fluids. These poisons are the real cancer, and they continue circulating unless a tumor filters them out. By destroying the tumor, the real cancer remains and keeps circulating until a new tumor is generated (called "recurrence"). By adding poisons in the form of chemotherapy drugs, antibiotics, immune-suppressants, etc., the real cancer (consisting of poisons) continues to spread and becomes ever more obstructive and aggressive. By removing the only outlet for these poisons, which is a tumor, the real cancer now begins to destroy the body. In other words, the treatment and neglecting to remove the real cancer (poisons) from the body are what kills the patient. Cancer cells don't endanger a person's life, but whatever causes them does. To repeat, cancer cells inside a tumor are harmless; and cutting out, burning or poisoning a tumor does not prevent the real cancer from spreading. Unless the real cancer is being addressed by cleansing the body and restoring normal digestive, eliminative functions, the growth of cancer cells continues to play an important role in the body's natural attempt to survive.

The body has to exert a lot more effort to maintain a tumor than to eliminate it. If it were not forced to use cancer growth as one of its last survival tactics, the body would not opt for this final attempt at self-preservation—final, because it could very well fail in its attempt to survive against the odds. As mentioned before, most tumors (about 90-95%) appear and disappear completely on their own, without any medical intervention. Millions of people walk around with cancers in their body and will never know they had them. There is no cancer treatment that can even remotely compete with the body's own healing mechanism, which we unfortunately label as disease. Cancer is not a disease; it is a very unusual, but apparently highly efficient, mechanism of survival and self-protection.

We ought to give the most developed and complex system in the universe—the human body—a little more credit than it has so far received, and trust that it knows perfectly well how to conduct its own affairs, even under the grimmest of circumstances.

The Body's Desperate Attempt to Live

Nobody wants to be attacked by anyone; this also applies to the cells of the body. Cells only go into a defensive mode and turn malignant if they need to ensure their own survival, at least for as long as they can. A spontaneous remission occurs when cells no longer need to defend themselves. Like every other disease, cancer is a toxicity crisis that, when allowed to come to its natural conclusion, will spontaneously relinquish its symptoms.

Of the 30 billion cells that a healthy body turns over each day, at least one percent are cancer cells. Does this mean, however, that all of us are destined to develop cancer—the disease? Certainly not. These cancer cells are products of a "programmed mutation" that keep our immune system alert, active, and stimulated.

The situation changes, though, when due to constant energy-depleting influences, the body can no longer deal adequately with the continual presence of worn-out, damaged, and cancerous cells. The result is a gradual build-up of congestion in the intercellular fluids. This can affect both the transportation of nutrients to the cells and the elimination of waste from the cells. Consequently, a large number of the corpses of dead cells begin to decompose, leaving behind a mass of degenerate protein fragments. To remove these harmful proteins, the body builds some of them into the basal membranes of the blood vessels and dumps the rest into the lymphatic ducts, which leads to lymphatic blockage. All of this disrupts the body's normal metabolic processes and alienates some groups of cells to such a degree that they become weak and damaged. Out of these cells, a number undergo genetic mutation and turn malignant. A cancerous tumor is born, and the toxicity crisis has reached its peak.

With the correct approaches, a tumor as big as an egg can spontaneously regress and disappear, regardless of whether it is in the brain, the stomach, a breast, or an ovary. The cure begins when the toxicity crisis stops. A toxicity crisis ends when we cease to deplete the body's energy (see Chapters Three and Four) and remove existing toxins from the blood, bile ducts, gastrointestinal tract, lymphatic vessels, and tissue fluids. Unless the body has been seriously damaged, it is perfectly capable of taking care of the rest. Medical intervention, on the other hand, reduces the possibility of a spontaneous remission to almost zero because of its suppressive and debilitating effects. Only those individuals with a strong physical and mental constitution can survive the treatment and heal themselves regardless.

Most cancers occur after a number of repeated warnings. These may include:

- Headaches that you continually stop with pain killers.[38]
- Tiredness that you keep suppressing with a cup of coffee, tea, or soda.
- Nervousness you try to control through nicotine.
- Medicines you take to ward off unwanted symptoms.
- Seasonal head colds, which you don't have time to let pass on their own.
- Not giving yourself enough time to relax, laugh, and be quiet.
- Conflicts that you keep avoiding.
- Pretending that you are always fine when you are not.
- Having a constant need to please others, while feeling unworthy and unloved by them.
- Possessing low self-confidence that makes you strive constantly to prove yourself to others.
- Rewarding yourself with comfort foods, because you feel undeserving.

All of these and similar symptoms are serious risk indicators for developing cancer or another illness.

There are no fundamental physiological differences between the development of a simple cold and the occurrence of a cancerous tumor. Both are attempts by the body to rid itself of accumulated toxins, but with varied degrees of intensity. Taking medical drugs in an attempt to ward off a head cold or an upper respiratory infection before giving your body the chance to eliminate the accumulated toxins, has a strongly suffocating effect on the cells of the body and a depressing effect on your self worth. It coerces the body to keep large amounts of cellular waste products, acidic substances, and, possibly, toxic drug chemicals in the tissue fluid (connective tissue) surrounding the cells. By

---

[38] Find out what causes pain and what happens when you suppress it in "Painkillers—The Beginning of a Vicious Cycle," Chapter Two of *Timeless Secrets of Health and Rejuvenation.*

repeatedly undermining the body's efforts to cleanse itself, the cells are increasingly shut off from their supply routes of oxygen and nutrients. This alters their basic metabolism and eventually affects the DNA molecule itself. The bottom line is, you are longer feeling yourself.

Located in the nucleus of every cell, the DNA makes use of its six billion genes to mastermind and control every single part and function of the body. Without the adequate supply of vital nutrients, the DNA has no choice but to alter its genetic program in order to guarantee the cell's survival. Mutated cells can survive in an environment of toxic waste. Soon they begin to draw nutrients from other surrounding cells. For these nutrient-deprived cells to survive, they also need to subject themselves to genetic mutation, which leads to the spreading or enlargement of the cancer. Cancerous growths are anaerobic, which means that they develop and survive without the use of oxygen.

Nobel Prize winner Dr. Otto Warburg was one of the first scientists to demonstrate the principal difference between a normal cell and a cancer cell. Both derive energy from glucose, but the normal cell utilizes oxygen to combine with the glucose, whereas the cancer cell breaks down glucose without the use of oxygen, yielding only 1/15 the energy per glucose molecule that the normal cell produces. It is very obvious that cancer cells opt for this relatively inefficient and unproductive method of obtaining energy because they no longer have access to oxygen. The capillaries supplying oxygen to a group of cells or to the connective tissue surrounding them (usually both) may be severely congested with harmful waste material, noxious substances such as food additives and chemicals, excessive proteins, or decomposing cellular debris. Thus, they are unable to deliver enough oxygen and nutrients.

Because their oxygen and nutrient supply is blocked, cancer cells have an insatiable appetite for sugar. This may also explain why people with constant cravings for sugary foods have a higher risk for developing cancer or why cancer patients often want to eat large amounts of sugar and sweets. The main waste product resulting from the anaerobic breakdown of glucose by cancer cells is lactic acid, which may explain why the body of a cancer patient is so acidic, in contrast to the naturally alkaline body of a healthy person.

To deal with the dangerously high levels of lactic acid and to find another source of energy, the liver reconverts some of the lactic acid into glucose. In doing so, the liver uses 1/5 the energy per glucose molecule that a normal cell can derive from it, but that's three times the energy a cancer cell will get from it. To help feed the cancer cells, the body even grows new blood vessels, funneling more and more sugar toward them. This means that the more the damaged cancer cells multiply, the less energy is available to the normal cells, hence the sugar cravings. In a toxic body, the concentrations of both oxygen and energy tend to be very low. This creates an environment where cancer spreads most easily. Unless the toxins and the cancer's food source are eliminated, and oxygen levels are sharply increased, the wasteful metabolism associated with cancer becomes self-sustaining and the cancer spreads further. If death occurs it is not caused by the cancer, though; it is due to the wasting of body tissues and final acidosis.

Genetic mutation is now believed to be the main **cause** of cancer; yet in truth it is only an **effect** of "cellular famine" and nothing more or less than the body's desperate, but often unsuccessful, attempt to live and survive. Something similar occurs in a person's body when he uses antibiotics to fight an infection. Most of the infection-causing bacteria that are being attacked by the antibiotics will be killed, but some of them will survive and reprogram their own genes to become antibiotic-resistant. Nobody really wants to die, and this includes bacteria.

The same law of nature applies to our body cells. *Cancer is the final attempt of the body to live, and not, as most people assume, to die.* Without gene mutation, those cells in the body that live in a toxic, anaerobic environment would simply suffocate and expire. Similar to bacteria that are attacked with antibiotics, many cells, in fact, succumb to the flood of toxins and die, but some manage to adjust to the abnormal changes of their natural environment. These cells know that they will eventually die, too, once their final survival tactics fail to keep the body alive.

To understand cancer and treat it more successfully than we currently do, we may have to radically alter our currently held views about it. We may also have to ask what its purpose is in the body and why the immune system fails to stop it from spreading. It is just not good enough to claim that cancer is an autoimmune disease that is out to kill the body. Such a notion (of the body trying to commit suicide) goes against the core principles of physical life. It makes so much more sense to say that cancer is nothing but the body's final attempt to live.

By removing all excessive waste from the gastrointestinal tract and any harmful deposits from the bile ducts, connective tissues, blood, and lymph vessels, the cancer cells will have no choice but to die or to reverse their faulty genetic program. Unless they are too damaged, they certainly can become normal, healthy cells again. Those anaerobic cells and seriously damaged cells that cannot make the adjustment to a clean, oxygenated environment may simply die off. By thoroughly cleansing the liver and gallbladder from gallstones and other toxins, the body's digestive power improves considerably, thereby increasing the production of digestive enzymes. Digestive and metabolic enzymes possess very powerful anti-tumor properties. When the body is being decongested through major cleansing and is given proper nourishment, these powerful enzymes have easy access to the cells of the body. Permanently damaged cells or tumor particles are easily and quickly neutralized and removed.

Many people in the world cure their own cancers in this fashion. Some are aware of this because their diagnosed tumors went into spontaneous remission without any form of medical treatment, but most will never even know they had cancer because they never received a diagnosis. After passing through a bout of the flu, a week of coughing up bad-smelling phlegm, or a couple of days with a high fever, many people eliminate massive amounts of toxins, and along with them, tumor tissue. Recent cancer research on gravely ill patients at M.D. Anderson Cancer Center in Houston, Texas revealed a promising treatment to kill cancer cells by giving them a cold, that is, injecting tumors with a cold virus. It may still take a while, though, before researchers discover that catching a few colds can do the same job. Thus, without interfering with the body's self-repair mechanisms, a person may experience a spontaneous remission of cancer, easily and with relatively minor discomfort.

Prostate Cancer and Its Risky Treatments

There is, indeed, enough scientific evidence to suggest that most cancers disappear by themselves if left alone. A 1992 Swedish study found that of 223 men who had early prostate cancer but did not receive *any* kind of medical treatment, only 19 died within ten years of diagnosis. Considering that one-third of men in the European Community have prostate cancer, but only one percent of them die (not necessarily from the cancer), it is very questionable to treat it at all. This is especially the case since research has revealed that treatment of the disease has not decreased mortality rates. On the contrary, survival rates are higher in groups of men whose "treatment" consists merely of watchful waiting, compared with groups undergoing prostate surgery. In the Trans-Urethral Resection Procedure (TURP), a 1/4-inch pipe is inserted into the penis to just below the base of the bladder, and the prostate is then fried with a hot wire loop. Far from being a safe procedure, one study found that a year after undergoing this surgery, 41% of the men had to wear diapers because of chronic leakage, and 88% were sexually impotent.

Even the screening procedure for prostate cancer can have serious consequences. According to a number of studies, more men who are screened with the PSA (prostate-specific-antigen) test die from prostate cancer than those who are not tested. A recent editorial in *The British Medical Journal* sized up the value of the PSA test with this comment: "At present the one certainty about PSA testing is that it causes harm." A high enough positive PSA test is typically followed by a prostate biopsy—a painful procedure that can result in bleeding and infection. Recent evidence suggests that a large number of these biopsies are completely unnecessary. In fact, they may be life-endangering. Each year, 98,000 people die in the U.S. because of medical testing errors, PSA tests included.

Another serious problem with PSA tests is that they are notoriously unreliable. In a 2003 study undertaken by the Memorial Sloan-Kettering Cancer Center in New York City, researchers found that half of the men with PSA levels high enough to be recommended for a biopsy had follow-up tests with normal PSA levels. In fact, doctors at the Fred Hutchinson Cancer Research Center (FHCRC) in Seattle estimated that PSA screening may result in an over-diagnosis rate of more than 40%. To make matters worse, a disturbing new study finds that fully 15% of older men whose PSA readings were considered perfectly normal had prostate cancer—some with relatively advanced tumors.

There is a much more reliable test than the PSA. The less well-known AMAS (Anti-Malignin Antibody Screening) blood test is very safe, inexpensive, and more than 95% accurate at detecting cancer of any type. Anti-Malignin antibody levels become elevated when any cancer cells are present in the body, and they can be detected several months before other clinical tests might find them. (Learn more about the AMAS test at the website Amascancertest.com.)

If men learned how to avoid a buildup of toxins in the body, prostate cancer could perhaps become the least common and least harmful of all cancers. Aggressive treatment of early prostate cancer is now a controversial issue, but it should be controversial for every type of cancer, at whatever stage of development; especially when simple approaches such as cleansing of the organs of elimination, a balanced, decongesting diet and regular exposure to sunlight can provide the body with what it needs to ward off cancer.

Avoid dairy products (except unsalted butter)
A Harvard study published in 1998 found a 50% increase in prostate cancer risk and a near doubling of risk of metastatic prostate cancer among men consuming high amounts of dairy products. The researchers attributed the high cancer risk from dairy consumption to the high total amount of calcium intake. High calcium levels in the body are known to increase the risk of cancer. Another Harvard study, published in October 2001, looked at dairy product intake among 20,885 men and found men

consuming the most dairy products had about 32% higher risk of developing prostate cancer than those consuming the least.

Excessive calcium intake may cause the following complications:

- Kidney stones
- Arthritic/joint and vascular degeneration
- Calcification of soft tissue
- Hypertension and stroke
- Elevated VLDL cholesterol
- Gastrointestinal disturbances
- Mood and depressive disorders
- Chronic fatigue
- Mineral deficiencies, including magnesium, zinc, iron and phosphorus
- Interference with vitamin D's cancer protective effects

About Prostrate Enlargement

Prescription drugs for an enlarged prostate encourage testosterone-to-estrogen conversion. This can greatly increase cancer risk. Men who take them have even grown female breasts. Also beware of estrogen-mimicking foods, including soy products and others, that both men and women are advised to eat. There are better ways to prevent prostate enlargement. In a study published in a recent issue of *The British Journal of Urology International*, researchers from the University of Chicago reviewed the results of nearly 20 trials that tested Permixon, a commercial extract of saw palmetto. The results were overwhelmingly positive, including improved urine flow; reduction of urinary urgency and pain; improved emptying of the bladder; reduction in size of the prostate gland after two years; and significant improvement in quality of life. In one trial, saw palmetto extract produced positive results similar to the drugs, but without the sexual dysfunction that accompanied drug use. Permixon is manufactured in Europe and not yet available in the U.S., but there are other supplements available here that are just as effective. Look for prostate products that contain beta-sitosterol, such as "Prostate Care" by *Healthy Choice Nutritionals,* which is even more powerful than saw palmetto.

Drinking 5 cups of green tea daily may slow prostate cancer growth, a Chinese study showed. The study was published online on October 7, 2003 in the *International Journal of Cancer* (Volume 108 Issue 1, pp. 130–135). More recent research (Japan Public Health Center-based Prospective study, 2007) showed that men could cut their risk of developing prostrate cancer by half. New research showed that black tea also has profound benefits in that it reduces prostate enlargement and prostate cancer in men who drink just 5 cups a week. Black tea may also prevent prostate cancer.

A powerful remedy consists of drinking the juice of broccoli that has been boiled in 16 to 20 ounces of water. Drink half of the juice on an empty stomach in the morning and the other half in the early evening. Repeat every day until cancer or prostate enlargement is gone. Results should be noticed within a week.

The product "Healthy Prostate & Ovary" is a blend of Chinese and Vietnamese herbs that are traditionally known to be supportive in promoting the health of ovary, prostate, breast and other organs and tissues. It also supports detoxification and production of energy, and enhances the body's immune response mechanisms. It contains extracts of Astragalus (root), Water Plaintain (root), *Crinum latifolium* (leaves), Bitter Melon (fruit), Papaya (leaves), and Soursop (leaves). Apparently Vietnamese men and women taking Crinum latifolium leaves rarely suffer from ailments of the reproductive system. In the U.S., this product is sold by NutriCology.com.

If red blotches appear on the penis, massage it with pure aloe vera gel, twice daily. Many prostate problems are due to trapped urinary deposits/crystals in the penis and disappear when removed by the gel. You should notice a clearing of the skin irritation within a few days.

For prostate enlargement I strongly recommend doing a series of liver flushes and one or several kidney cleanses.[39]

---

[39] For step-by-step instructions, see *The Amazing Liver and Gallbladder Flush.*

Why Most Cancers Disappear Naturally

Every toxicity crisis, from a complex cancer to a simple head cold, is actually a healing crisis that, when supported by cleansing measures, leads to a swift recovery. However, if interfered with by symptom-suppressive measures, a usually short-lived "recovery" may easily turn into a chronic disease condition. Unfortunately, cancer researchers do not dare or do not care to find a natural cure for cancer; this is not what they are trained and paid for. Even if they did stumble over a natural cure, it would never be made public.

Rose Papac, M.D., a professor of oncology at Yale University School of Medicine, once pointed out that there is little opportunity these days to see what happens to cancers if left untreated. "Everyone feels impelled to treat immediately when they see these diseases," says Papac, who has studied cases of spontaneous remissions of cancer. Being stifled with fear, and in some cases being paranoid about finding a quick-acting remedy for the dreaded illness, many people don't give their body the chance to cure itself, but instead choose to destroy what does not need to be destroyed. This may be one of the main reasons spontaneous remissions occur in so few cancer patients nowadays.

On the other hand, numerous researchers have reported over the years that various conditions such as typhoid fever, coma, menopause, pneumonia, chickenpox and even hemorrhage can spark spontaneous remissions of cancer. However, official explanations of how these remissions relate to the disappearance of the cancer are non-existent. Because they are unexplained phenomena, seemingly having no scientific basis, they are not used for further cancer research. Consequently, the scientific community's interest in discovering the mechanism for how the body cures itself of cancer remains almost non-existent. These "miracle cures" seem to happen most frequently in certain types of malignancies: kidney cancer, melanoma (cancer of the skin), lymphomas (cancers of the lymph), and neuroblastoma (a nerve cell cancer that affects infants).

Considering that most of the body's organs have eliminative

functions, it stands to reason that liver, kidney, colon, lung, lymph, and skin cancers are more likely to disappear when these major organs and systems of elimination are no longer over-loaded with toxins. Likewise, malignant tumors do not develop in a healthy body with intact defense and repair functions. They only thrive in a specific internal environment that encourages and promotes their growth. Cleansing such an environment, by whatever means, can make a tremendous difference with regard to healing cancer.

A toxicity crisis like pneumonia or chickenpox, unless sup-pressed or combated, removes large amounts of toxins and helps the cells to "breathe" freely again. Fever, sweat, loss of blood, mucus discharge, diarrhea, and vomiting are additional outlets for toxins to leave the body. After breaking down and removing the toxins in an unhindered way, the immune system receives a natural and much-needed boost. A renewed immune stimulation based on reduced overall toxicity in the body can be sufficient to do away with a malignant tumor that no longer has a role to play in the survival of the body. The undesirable chickenpox, pneu-monia, fever, or other such symptoms may actually be "a gift from God" (to use another unscientific expression) that could save a person's life. Refusing to accept the gift could cost the ill person his life. Many people die unnecessarily because they are prevented from going through all the phases of an illness. Illnesses are nothing other than the body's many attempts to create outlets for trapped poisonous substances. Blocking the exit routes for these poisons, which happens when symptoms are being treated away, can suffocate the body and stop its vital functions. The body has an innate tendency and capacity to heal itself. Medical treatment should be limited to supporting the body in this effort rather than interfering with it. The current medical model is based on suppression and intervention, not on assistance and support. This principle applies especially to modern vaccina-tion programs and other rarely considered factors.

Chapter Five

Other Major Cancer Risks

Vaccinations—Ticking Time Bombs?

The suppression of children's diseases through unnatural immunization programs can put the children at high risk for eventually developing cancer. Chickenpox, measles, and other natural self-immunization programs (wrongly called "childhood diseases") help endow a child's immune system with the ability to counteract potential disease-causing agents more efficiently and without having to go through a major toxicity crisis.

With more than 550,000 annual cancer deaths in the United States alone, the justification for mandatory immunization programs in this country is highly questionable. The standard approach to establishing immunity, which is unproved and unscientific, may undermine and override the body's own far superior programs of self-immunization. The body gains natural immunity through exposure to pathogens and, occasionally, a healing crisis, which naturally eliminates cancer-producing toxins. Vaccines, on the other hand, suppress natural immunity and replace it with fake immunity.

By design, all vaccines depress immune functions. The cocktail of toxic chemicals and metals, the viruses, and the foreign DNA/RNA from animal tissues in the vaccines impair the immune system. Many of the vaccines contain neurotoxins and actual carcinogens. This is what is being pumped into a healthy body: aluminum, thirmersol, formaldehyde, carbolic acid (phenol), the antibiotics neomycin, streptomycin and a variety of other drugs, the solvent acetone, glycerin (which can cause death), sodium hydroxide, sorbitol, hydrolyzed gelatin, benzethonium chloride, methylparaben and other chemicals known or suspected of causing cancer. (Conscious Rasta Report vol. 3, no. 9: *Epidemic*.)

The vaccines especially reduce polymorphonuclear neutro-

145

phils (PMNs)[40], lymphocyte viability, neutrophil hyper-segmentation, and white cell count—all essential factors for maintaining a normal, healthy immune system and, thus, keeping track of daily cell mutations. It is insane to sacrifice naturally acquired immunity with a state of temporary, incomplete immunity against one or several diseases, including innocuous childhood diseases.

Vaccines also rob the body of vital immune-enhancing nutri-ents, like vitamin C, A and zinc, which are essential to build or have a strong immune system. The poisons contained in vaccines don't allow a young child to develop a healthy immune system, which makes it susceptible to many illnesses in the future. So are there safe vaccines?

"The only safe vaccine is the one that is never used." ~ James Shannon, former National Institutes of Health (NIH) Director. Children are the most vulnerable because their immune systems are practically defenseless against the poisons in the vaccines. They have a lot against them since their mothers are **not** passing on immunity to them in the breast milk (because they were vaccinated and no longer make antibodies). Children die at a rate eight times faster than normal after a DPT shot. James R. Shannon of NIH understood this when he said "No vaccination can be proven safe before it is given to children."

"I haven't got a flu shot and I don't intend to." ~ George W. Bush, 2004 Presidential Candidate and President. Does Mr. Bush know more than the rest of us?

Researchers at the University of Chicago Medical Center say that 98 million Americans who took polio shots in the 1950s and 1960s may get a deadly brain cancer from the inoculations.

Whether manufactured vaccines directly or indirectly cause cancer is irrelevant. It is important to know, however, that conventional immunization programs can prevent the body from developing a potentially life-saving healing crisis. All these different vaccines administered to millions of children and adults every year profoundly affect the body's ability to heal itself. The injected vaccines contain large protein molecules that clog up the

---

[40] PMNs are our body's defenses against pathogenic bacteria and viruses.

lymphatic vessels and lymph nodes, and cause metabolic waste products and turned-over, dead cells to become trapped in the tissue fluids. The same effect undermines the efficacy of immune cells circulating in the lymph.

For detailed information about what vaccines can do to the human body and the health of the population, check out my free published articles "Vaccination Programs under Scrutiny," parts 1-3, www.naturalnews.com/Author206.html, or read Chapter Thirteen, Eight Dangerous Myths of Modern Living, *Timeless Secrets of Health and Rejuvenation.* To remove harmful chemicals and toxic metals from the body, I recommend using the zeolite product, Natural Cellular Defense from Waiora, MMS, and marine phytoplankton. (See more information at www.ener-chi.com.)

Wearing Bras Impairs Lymph Drainage

There are other factors that affect proper lymph drainage and circulation. Regularly wearing a bra impairs the proper flow of lymph and may greatly increase the chance of developing breast cancer. Researcher David Moth conducted an experiment in which he measured the actual pressure exerted by bras on the underlying lymphatic ducts. He says, "The results suggest that the lightest possible bras will still exert pressures in excess of that found within the lymphatic vessels." Several other studies confirm the link between bra wearing and breast cancer. In 1991, C. Hsieh and D. Trichopoulos studied breast size and left/right handedness as risk factors for breast cancer. They noted in their findings that premenopausal women who do not wear a bra had less than half the risk of breast cancer than did their bra-wearing peers. This study was published in the *European Journal of Cancer*, 1991;27(2):131-5.

Another more recent study (2000), published in *Chronobiology International* (the journal of biological and medical rhythm research), found that wearing a bra decreased melatonin production and increased the core body temperature. Melatonin is a powerful antioxidant and hormone that promotes good sleep, fights aging, boosts the immune system, and slows the growth of certain types of cancer, including breast cancer.

The most comprehensive studies on this subject were performed by the husband and wife team of applied medical anthropologists, Sydney Ross Singer and Soma Grismaijer. Singer and Grismaijer found that the Maoris, the indigenous people of New Zealand who integrated into western culture, had the same rates of breast cancer as their western peers. The marginalized aboriginals of Australia, interestingly, had practically no breast cancer. The same was true for westernized Japanese, Fijians, and women from other cultures who converted to the practice of bra wearing; when they did so, their rates of breast cancer soared.

In the early 1990s Singer and Grismaijer studied the bra-wearing habits of 4,500 women in five cities across the U.S. They found that 3 out of 4 women who wore their bras 24 hours per day developed breast cancer. Among those who wore their bras more than 12 hours per day but not to bed, 1 out of 7 developed breast cancer. This is a slightly higher cancer rate than the standard female population of 1 in 8. By comparison, merely 1 out of 152 women who wore their bras less than 12 hours per day had breast cancer, and only 1 out of 168 women who wore bras rarely or never developed cancer of the breast. In other words, women who wore a bra 24 hours per day were 125 times more likely to develop breast cancer than women who rarely or never wore a bra. Interestingly, women who chose to go braless had the same breast cancer rates as men did!

The Early Puberty and Breast Cancer Link

Girls in the United States and other modern countries are reaching puberty at very early ages, which has been shown to increase their risk of breast cancer. Just decades ago, biological signs of female puberty—menstruation, breast development, and growth of pubic and underarm hair—typically occurred around 13 years of age or older. And in the early twentieth century it was more like 16 or 17. Today, girls as young as eight are increasingly showing these signs. Apparently, African-American girls are particularly vulnerable to early puberty. Even five and six year olds now go through precocious puberty (aka early sexual development). Early puberty exposes girls to more estrogen—a major risk for hormone–related breast cancers. According to data published by biologist Sandra Steingraber, girls who have their first menstrual period before age 12 have a 50 percent higher risk of developing breast cancer than those who begin menstruating at age 16. "For every year we could delay a girl's first menstrual period," she says, "we could prevent thousands of breast cancers."

Potential causes for this trend include rising childhood obesity rates and inactivity, cows' milk- and soy-infant formulas, bovine growth hormones commonly added to milk, hormones and antibiotics in beef, and non-fermented soy products, such as soy milk and tofu, which mimic estrogens. Soy's estrogenic effects exceed those produced by the birth control pill by 4 to 5 times. (Also see Soy and Cancer below.) Other causes may include bisphenol A and phthalates (found in many plastics, such as baby containers, water bottles, and the inner lining of soda cans), other man-made chemicals that affect hormonal balance (such as those found in cosmetics, toothpastes, shampoos, and hair dyes), stress at home and at school, and excessive TV viewing and media use.

Soy—A Carcinogen for Humans?

The food industry, which operates in a similar way to the pharmaceutical industry, has successfully convinced the population that soy is a health food. Soy has even been praised as the miracle food that will save the world from starvation. Soy supporters claim it can provide an ideal source of protein, lower cholesterol, protect against cancer and heart disease, alleviate menopause symptoms, and prevent osteoporosis. However, when you look beyond the propaganda, the facts about soy paint a very different picture. In spite of soy's impressive nutritional content, soy products are biologically useless to the body, for reasons explained below. Today, soy is contained in thousands of different food products, which has led to a massive escalation of disease in both developed and underdeveloped countries.

Given the fact that soybeans are grown on farms that use toxic, cancer-producing pesticides and herbicides—and many are from genetically engineered plants[41]—increasing evidence suggests soy is a major health hazard. With a few exceptions, such as miso, tempeh and other carefully fermented soy products, soy is not suitable for human consumption. Eating soy, soy milk, and regular tofu increases risks of serious health conditions. In addition, soy is a common food allergen. Numerous studies have found that soy products:

- increase the risk of breast cancer in women, brain damage in both men and women, and abnormalities in infants
- contribute to thyroid disorders, especially in women
- promote kidney stones (because of excessively high levels of oxalates which combine with calcium in the kidneys)
- weaken the immune system
- cause severe, potentially fatal food allergies
- accelerate brain weight loss in aging users

Soy products contain:

- Phytoestrogens (isoflavones) genistein and daidzein, which mimic and sometimes block the hormone estrogen.
- Phytic acids, which reduce the absorption of many vitamins and minerals, including calcium, magnesium, iron, and zinc, thereby causing mineral deficiencies.
- "Antinutrients" or enzyme inhibitors that inhibit enzymes needed for protein digestion and amino acid uptake.
- Haemaggluttin, which causes red blood cells to clump together and inhibits oxygen uptake and growth.
- Trypsin inhibitors that can cause pancreatic enlargement and, eventually, cancer.

---

[41] In the U.S., 80% of all soy beans come from genetically engineered soy plants.

Phytoestrogens are potent anti-thyroid agents which are present in vast quantities in soy. Infants exclusively fed on a soy-based formula have 13,000 to 22,000 times more estrogen compounds in their blood than babies fed a milk-based formula. This would be the estrogenic equivalent of at least five birth control pills per day. For this reason, premature development of girls (early puberty) has been linked to the use of soy formula, as has the underdevelopment of males. Infant soy formula and soy milk have been linked to autoimmune-thyroid disease, and now also to death.

In 2007, two parents were convicted of murder and given life sentences in prison for starving their 6-week-old baby to death by feeding it with soy milk and apple juice. Now, soy experts are again calling for clear and proper warning labels on all soy milk products—following this and several other babies' hospitalizations or deaths under similar circumstances.

Only soy products, such as miso, tempeh and natto, provide soy nutrients that can easily be absorbed and utilized by the body. To make soy products nutritious and healthy, they must be carefully fermented—according to the traditional preparation methods used in Japan. Typically, soy must be fermented for at least two summers, ideally for 5-6 years, before it becomes beneficial for the body.

A recent study of 700 elderly Indonesians showed that properly fermented soy, such as tempeh, miso, natto and soybean sprouts (not genetically modified), helped improve memory, particularly in participants over 68 years of age. The study also affirms that high tofu consumption (at least once a day) was associated with worse memory, particularly among those over age 68. The study was published in *Dementia and Geriatric Cognitive Disorders*, June 27, 2008; 26(1):50-57. If you want to avoid dementia, avoid all processed soy milks, tofu, soy burgers, soy ice cream, soy cheese, and all other soy-containing junk foods.

In spite of the documented scientific evidence that shows non-fermented soy to be carcinogenic and also cause DNA and chromosome damage, the multi-billion dollar soy industry has managed to turn this generally worthless food into one of the most widely used "nutritious foods" of all times. In a written statement, a spokesman for *Protein Technologies* said that they had ". . . teams of lawyers to crush dissenters, could buy scientists to give evidence, owned television channels and newspapers, could divert medical schools and could even influence governments . . ."

Lipid specialist and nutritionist Mary Enig, PhD explains one of the main reasons behind the soy revolution. She says, "The reason there's so much soy in America is because they [the soy industry] started to plant soy to extract the oil from it and soy oil became a very large industry. Once they had as much oil as they did in the food supply, they had a lot of soy protein residue left over, and since they can't feed it to animals, except in small amounts, they had to find another market." In other words, the human population became an effective garbage dumpster for the food industry, while making the medical industry increasingly profitable as a result of treating the many soy-caused illnesses. This is not unlike the pouring of the poison fluoride—a hazardous waste product from aluminum plants—into the municipal water to "save" children from developing bad teeth. To dispose of fluoride in any other way would be extremely costly.

Animals that naturally ferment their foods in their stomach before absorbing them can break down the enzyme inhibitors soy contains and, thus, make use of the proteins. Not all foods that grow on this planet are beneficial for human beings. In fact, animals inhabited the planet long before humans did; therefore, most foods were actually designed to feed and sustain the animal kingdom. The recent additon of large amounts of non-fermented soy in the human food chain has already had disastrous consequences on the health of millions of people and will continue to do so unless the masses educate themselves about the deceptive practices of the food industry and the government agencies that are supposed to protect us from harm.

Why French Fries can Cause Cancer

French fries and other fried, baked, or roasted carbohydrate-rich foods contain the chemical acrylamide, which has been implicated to be a human carcinogen. Women who eat approximately one portion of chips a day may drastically double their risk of ovarian and endometrial cancer (cancer of the uterus lining), according to a new study published in the journal *Cancer Epidemiology, Biomarkers & Prevention.*

Acrylamide was accidentally discovered in foods in April 2002 by scientists in Sweden when they found large amounts of the chemical in potato chips, French fries and bread that had been heated at temperatures above 120 degrees Centigrade (250 degrees Fahrenheit). Prior to that, acrylamide was believed to be a solely industrial chemical. The production of acrylamide in the heating process was shown to be clearly temperature-dependent. Over-cooking and microwaving foods may also produce large amounts of acrylamide. Boiled and unheated foods don't contain acrylamide.

In this new study, researchers examined data gathered by the Netherlands Cohort study on diet and cancer occurrence among 62,573 women. The women who ingested the most acrylamide, 40.2 micrograms per day, had a 29 percent higher risk of endometrial cancer and a 78 percent higher risk of ovarian cancer. Surprisingly, women who had never smoked had a 99 percent higher risk of endometrial cancer and a 122 percent higher risk of ovarian cancer among those with the highest acrylamide intake.

The March 15, 2005 issue of the *Journal of the American Medical Association* (JAMA) contained an article entitled "Acrylamide Intake and Breast Cancer Risk in Swedish Women," written by Lorelei A. Mucci, ScD, MPH. The study cohort consisted of 43,404 Swedish women in the Women's Lifestyle and Health Cohort. The women's greatest single source of acrylamide was from coffee (54% of intake), fried potatoes (12% of intake), and crisp bread (9% of intake).

Electric Light and Cancer

As explained before, a strong link exists between low levels of the hormone melatonin and cancer. Melatonin protects genetic material from mutation, according to Russell Reiter, professor of cellular and structural biology at the University of Texas. "Night light suppresses the body's production of melatonin and thus can increase the risk of cancer-related mutations," he told a gathering in London. Scott Davis, chairman of the department of epidemiology at the University of Washington, stated that "while the link between light at night and cancer may seem like a stretch on the surface, there is an underlying biological basis for it." Both Davis and Reiter have been studying how night lighting affects the production of female hormones, which, in turn, can affect the risk of breast cancer. "We have found a relationship between light at night and night-shift work to breast cancer risk," Davis said. "The studies indicate that night work disrupts the activity of melatonin, which leads to excessive production of hormones in women." Melatonin, which is produced at around 9:30 p.m. and reaches peak level secretions at around 1:00 a.m., also controls a powerful gene that ensures cells don't live beyond their normal lifespan. If they liver longer than they should, they become cancerous.

The message here is to get at least eight hours of sleep every day, starting before 10 p.m. Shut off or block out any artificial lighting around you. In addition, as explained before, get regular exposure to sunlight without using sunglasses and sunscreen lotions. These are two of the most effective measures for the treatment and prevention of cancer.

Air Pollution and Stress in Cities

As reported by NaturalNews.com in May 2008, a Canadian study has shown that women with breasts composed of 25 percent or more dense tissue have five times the breast cancer of women with fattier breasts. The study also found that women with dense breasts were 18 times more likely to have a breast tumor detected within one year of a negative mammogram.

Now, recent research conducted by the Princess Grace Hospital in London (U.K.) and presented to the Radiological Society of North America showed that women who live and work in cities have a significantly higher risk of developing breast cancer than women who live in the country. To determine the reasons for this occurrence, researchers examined the breast tissue of 972 British women between the ages of 45 and 54. They found that the breasts of women who were living and working in cities were more than twice as likely to have 25 percent or more dense tissue.

Researchers hypothesized that city dwellers may have increased breast density because of hormone-disrupting toxins contained in air pollution. They also cited stress as a possible factor.

I might add that the forceful mammogram procedure could also contribute to breast cancers in women with denser breast tissue, by injuring it. Softer, fattier breast tissue can tolerate the potentially injurious mammography screening much better.

Microwave Ovens

Do you ever wonder what microwaves do to water, food, and your body? Russian researchers have found decreased nutritional value, cancer-making compounds, and brain-damaging *radiolytics* in virtually all microwave-prepared foods. Eating microwave-prepared meals can also cause loss of memory and concentration, emotional instability, and a decline in intelligence, according to the research. In studying the nutritional value of foods cooked with microwaves, the Russian scientists found significant dimming of their "vital energy field." This was noted in up to 90% of all microwave-prepared foods.

In addition, the B complex, C, and E vitamins linked with stress-reduction and the prevention of cancer and heart disease—as well as the essential trace minerals needed for optimum brain and body functioning—were rendered useless by microwaves, even at short cooking durations. Microwave-cooked food is reduced to the nutritional equivalent of cardboard. If you do not want to develop nutrient deficiencies, you may be better off removing this appliance from your kitchen. In addition, all microwave ovens have unavoidable leakages. Hence, the radiation accumulates in the kitchen furniture, becoming a source of radiation in itself.

Microwave usage in the preparation of food leads to lymphatic disorders and an inability to protect the body against certain cancers. The research found increased rates of cancer cell formation in the blood of people eating microwave-cooked meals. The Russians also reported increased rates of stomach and intestinal cancers, more digestive and excretive disorders, and a higher percentage of cell tumors, including sarcoma.

The Germans were the first to use microwave technology in the 1930s. At the beginning of the Second World War, German scientists developed a radar system based on technically generated microwaves. During the extremely cold wintertime, soldiers gathered around the radar screens to get warm, but they developed blood cancers. Subsequently, the German army abandoned the use of radar. However, after German scientists learned that microwaves heated human tissue, they thought these waves could also heat food, and so they invented the microwave oven with the intention to provide German soldiers with warm meals during the battles against the Soviet Union. However, the soldiers who ate foods heated in microwave ovens also developed cancers of the blood, just like the radar technicians. As a result of this discovery, the use of microwave ovens was banned in the entire Third Reich.

Are microwaves any safer today than they were 80 years ago? Certainly not; they are the same microwaves. Microwaves rip apart the molecular bonds that make food the nourishing substance that it is. Microwave ovens hurl high-frequency microwaves that boil the moisture within food and its packaging by whipsawing water molecules dizzyingly back-and-forth at more than a billion reversals per second. This frantic friction fractures food molecules, rearranging their chemical composition into weird new configurations unrecognizable as food by the human body. By destroying the molecular structures of food, the body cannot help but turn the food into waste—not harmless

156

waste, but "nuclear waste."

Other Side effects of microwave exposure include:
- High blood pressure
- Adrenal exhaustion
- Heart disease
- Migraines
- Dizziness
- Memory loss
- Disconnected thoughts
- Attention disorders
- Brain damage
- Anxiety
- Increased crankiness
- Depression
- Sleep disturbance
- Stomach pain
- Appendicitis
- Cataracts
- Hair loss
- Reproductive disorders

Eating microwave-damaged foods can lead to a considerable stress response in the body and, thereby, alter the blood chemistry. For example, eating organic vegetables zapped by microwaves will send your cholesterol soaring. According to Swiss scientist Dr. Hans U. Hertel, "Blood cholesterol levels are less influenced by cholesterol content of the food than by stress factors." While the Russian government banned microwave ovens in 1976 for a very good reason, these appliances play a prominent role in the daily cooking routines at 9 out of 10 American homes.

Reporting for the Forensic Research Document of Agricultural and Resource Economics (AREC), William P. Kopp now states: "The effects of microwaved food byproducts are long-term, permanent within the human body. Minerals, vitamins, and nutrients of all microwaved food is reduced or altered so that the human body gets little or no benefit, or the human body absorbs altered compounds that cannot be broken down."

Microwaves turn healthy food into deadly poison. Seeing the unprecedented cancer epidemic in the U.S. and other countries that largely rely on microwaves for cooking foods, it may be wise if we followed the example of the former Russian Federation and the Third Reich, at least in this respect, and stopped using microwave ovens altogether.

Dehydration

Cancer growth usually occurs in areas of severe dehydration. Many people suffer from dehydration without being aware of it. Dehydration is a condition in which body cells do not receive enough water for basic metabolic processes. The cells can run dry for a number of reasons:

- Lack of water intake (anything less than six glasses of pure water per day)
- Regular consumption of beverages that have diuretic effects, e.g. coffee, caffeinated tea, carbonated beverages, such as soda pop, and alcohol, including beer and wine
- Regular consumption of stimulating foods or substances, such as meat, hot spices, chocolate, sugar, tobacco, narcotic drugs, soda pop, artificial sweeteners, and the like
- Stress
- Taking any of a number of pharmacological drugs
- Excessive exercise
- Overeating and excessive weight gain
- Watching television daily for several hours

Any of these factors have a blood-thickening effect and, thereby, force cells to give up water. The cellular water is used to restore blood thinness. To avoid self-destruction, however, the cells begin to hold onto water. They do this by increasing the thickness of their membranes. The clay-like substance, cholesterol, starts to envelope the cells and, thereby, prevents loss of cellular water. Although this emergency measure may preserve water and save the cell's life for the time being, it also reduces the cell's ability to absorb new water, as well as much-needed nutrients. Subsequently, some of the unabsorbed water and nutrients accumulate in the connective tissues surrounding the cells, causing swelling of the body and water retention in the legs, kidneys, face, eyes, arms, and other parts. This leads to considerable weight gain. At the same time, the blood plasma and lymph fluids become thickened and congested. Dehydration also affects the natural fluidity of bile, thereby promoting the formation of gallstones. All of these factors combined are sufficient to trigger the survival mechanism of cell mutation.

Tea, coffee, carbonated beverages, and chocolate share the same nerve toxin and stimulant: *caffeine*. Caffeine, which is readily released into the blood, triggers a powerful immune response that helps to counteract and eliminate this irritant. The toxic irritant stimulates the adrenal glands, and to some extent, the body's many cells, to release the stress hormones, adrenaline and cortisol, into the bloodstream. The resulting sudden surge in energy is commonly referred to as "the fight or flight response." If consumption of stimulants continues on a regular basis, however, this natural defense response of the body becomes overused and ineffective. The almost constant secretion of stress hormones, which are highly toxic compounds in and of themselves, eventually alters the blood chemistry and causes damage to the immune, endocrine, and nervous systems. Future defense responses are weakened, and the body becomes more prone to infections and other ailments, including cell mutation.

The boost in energy experienced after drinking a cup of coffee is not a direct result of the caffeine itself; rather, the immune system's attempt get rid of it provides the effect. However, an overexcited and suppressed immune system eventually fails to provide the "energizing" adrenaline and cortisol boosts needed to free the body from the acidic nerve toxin, caffeine. At this stage, people say that they are "used" to a stimulant, such as coffee. They tend to increase their intake of it to feel the "benefits." The often-heard expression, "I am dying for a cup of coffee," reflects the true peril of their situation.

Since the body's cells continuously have to give up some of

their own water for the removal of the nerve toxin *caffeine*, regular consumption of coffee, tea, or sodas causes them to become dehydrated. For every cup of tea or coffee a person ingests, the body has to mobilize about 2-3 cups of water just to remove the caffeine, a luxury it cannot afford. This also applies to soft drinks, pharmaceutical drugs, or any other substance or activity that brings about the release of stress hormones, including watching TV for many hours. As a rule, all stimulants have a strong dehydrating effect on the bile, blood, and digestive juices. To heal a cancerous growth, stimulants are counterproductive, and it is best to avoid them.

To prevent dehydration, be certain to drink about 6-8 glasses of water (filtered and not chilled) per day.

If you have cancer, also avoid:

Chlorinated water: One of the most powerful cancer-producing chemicals around. Avoid drinking unfiltered tap water, swimming in chlorinated pools, or showering without a chlorine-removing filter. (You absorb more chlorine through the skin than you could possibly ingest from drinking tap water.)

Fluoride in municipal drinking water: Just as carcinogenic as chlorine. Fluoride actually increases your body's uptake of aluminum. Use a water filter that takes out fluoride.

Electromagnetic radiation: Electromagnetic radiation interferes with the body's own electromagnetic field and undermines basic intercellular communication. Remove all electrical appliances or equipment from the bedroom, including electric blankets and electric alarm clocks. By placing a larger Ionized Stone (see Other Products and Services by the Author at the end of the book) in, above, or below the fuse box in your house, many of the harmful effects of electromagnetic radiation are nullified.

Wireless devices, as explained in Chapter Four.

Pesticides and other chemical toxins as found in non-organic foods, conventional household cleaning products, commercial

160

beauty products, hair dyes (see information below), shampoos, skin lotions, and other personal care products, overtax and suppress the immune system when all its energy and resources are needed to heal the cancer. Especially avoid cosmetics with aluminum bases, mineral powders that contain bismuth, and aluminum-laden antiperspirants which are known to increase the risk of developing Alzheimer's disease by as much as 300%!

Hair dye: The fact that hairdressers have the highest rate of breast cancer of any profession prompted researchers to study the link between hair dye and cancer. A number of different studies found that women who use hair dye at least once a month are twice as likely to develop bladder cancer as those who do not. The risk triples when women use hair dye regularly for 15 or more years. These risks are the same regardless whether the women use permanent, semi-permanent, or rinse applications. The chemicals contained in commercial hair dye products penetrate the scalp and enter the blood stream. The kidneys filter them out and pass them into the urinary bladder where they damage the cells of the bladder, leading to repeated bladder infections and cell mutation.

To minimize the harm from hair dyes, make certain to drink enough water each day (6-8 glasses), cleanse your kidneys and the liver on a regular basis (see directions in *The Amazing Liver and Gallbladder Flush*), choose foiling and highlights, natural plant-based Henna dyes, or plant-based dyes, such as from Aveda and Herbatint.

Arsenic, asbestos, and **nickel,** since these can cause lung and other cancers. You wouldn't think that arsenic is something you would ingest somehow, unless someone intended to poison you. Well, if you eat chicken, you actually get a lot arsenic into your body. The poultry industry loves arsenic because it acts as a massive growth stimulant. Dr. Ellen Silbergeld, a researcher from the Johns Hopkins School of Public Health, commented about the industry's practice of using arsenic compounds in its feed: "It's an issue everybody is trying to pretend doesn't exist." Yet inorganic arsenic exposure is a known risk factor for diabetes mellitus. It is also considered one of the prominent environmental causes of cancer mortality in the world. If you have prostate cancer or don't want to develop it, avoid eating chicken.

Benzene, which can cause leukemia, and **formaldehyde** which can cause nasal and nasopharyngeal cancer. Formaldehyde is commonly used in the production of more complex chemicals, such as polymers and resins. Resins are used in adhesives, such as those found in plywood and carpeting. Formaldehyde is also used in sanitary paper products, such as facial tissue, table napkins, and roll towels. Most insulation material, moulded products, and paints contain formaldehyde derivatives, too.

Environmental/food toxins: Many babies are born toxic due to the toxic load of their mothers. Blood samples from newborns contained an average of **287 toxins**, including **mercury, fire retardants, pesticides** and **Teflon** chemicals, according to a 2004 study by the Environmental Working Group (EWG).

Teflon: This chemical in cooking pots is also carcinogenic. Food should never be prepared in Teflon cookware. Use glass, cast iron, carbon steel, titanium, and enamel cookware.

PVC shower curtains: They emit a strong smell and can cause serious damage to your liver as well as to the nervous, reproductive, and respiratory systems. The smell comes from deadly chemicals, including toluene, ethylbenzene, phenol, methyl isobutyl ketone, xylene, acetophenone, and cumene, all named dangerous air pollutants by the EPA. Polyvinyl chloride (PVC) shower curtains are sold at Kmart, Bed Bath & Beyond, Wal-Mart, Sears, and Target. "One of the curtains tested released measurable quantities of as many as 108 volatile organic compounds into the air, some of which persisted for nearly a month," according to a recent *New York Sun* article. To be safe, replace your PVC curtains with cloth curtains or glass doors.

Artificial sweeteners such as aspartame and Splenda: Once in the body, they break down into powerful carcinogenic compounds.[42]

Alcohol consumption: It causes liver bile duct congestion, suppresses the immune system and reduces magnesium in the

---

[42] For details about the effects of artificial sweeteners, see *Timeless Secrets of Health and Rejuvenation.*

body—all risks for developing cancer.[43] In 2002, the *British Journal of Cancer* reported that 4 percent of all breast cancers in the United Kingdom—about 44,000 cases a year—are due to alcohol consumption. And, according to findings presented in San Diego at the 2008 annual meeting of the American Association for Cancer Research, alcohol, consumed even in small amounts, may significantly increase the risk of breast cancer—particularly estrogen-receptor/progesterone-receptor positive breast cancer. The study followed more than 184,000 postmenopausal women for an average of seven years. Those women who had less than one drink per day had a 7 percent increased risk of breast cancer compared to those who did not drink at all. Women who drank 1-2 drinks a day had a 32 percent increased risk, and those who had three or more glasses of alcohol a day had up to a 51 percent increased risk. The risk was seen mostly in those 70 percent of tumors classified as estrogen receptor- and progesterone receptor-positive. The study showed no difference in risks whether women consumed beer, wine, or hard liquor.

Growth hormones in cow's milk: Samuel Epstein, M.D., a scientist at the University of Illinois School of Public Health, points out that rBGH milk is "supercharged with high levels of a natural growth factor (IGF-1), excess levels of which have been incriminated as major causes of breast, colon, and prostate cancers."

Synthetic vitamins: Manufactured vitamins (non-methylated, inexpensive junk vitamins) can rob your body of energy and actually cause the vitamin deficiencies you want to avoid by taking these vitamins. Natural vitamins as found in fruits and vegetables, on the other hand, **donate** energy to your cells.

Synthetic vitamin pills contain as much as 90% pure filler. The absorption rate of these vitamins is often less than 5%.

---

[43] A Swedish study showed that women with the highest magnesium intake had a 40 per cent lower risk of developing cancer than those with the lowest intake of the mineral. And researchers from the School of Public Health at the University of Minnesota found that diets rich in magnesium reduced the occurrence of colon cancer.

Taking many vitamin supplements can also greatly burden the digestive system, liver and kidneys. Besides, it is virtually impossible to produce vitamin products that have the right balance between the various vitamins they contain. Each person's vitamin requirement is uniquely different and it changes all the time; therefore, no vitamin product can ever match and meet that requirement. Leaving it up to the body to decide how many vitamins to extract from the foods, is the only really safe way to ingest them.

It is always best to get your vitamins from the foods you eat. Vitamins are naturally toxic, acidic, and reactive. Fruits and vegetables contain natural, neutralizing agents to keep the vitamins from causing harm in the body. Even a high quality methylated vitamin (one that uses the coenzyme of the vitamin), is stripped of these agents and can trigger an imbalanced response by the body, such as irritation and removing existing vitamins (thereby causing a vitamin deficiency). For detailed information about the "Hidden Perils of Vitamin Pills," see Chapter 14 of *Timeless Secrets of Health and Rejuvenation.*

Grilling meat, poultry or fish: In April 2008 the American Institute of Cancer Research urged everyone to rethink the pastime of barbecuing meat. After analyzing the results of 7,000 studies, the Institute concluded that grilling any meat—whether red, white or fish—creates potent cancer-producing chemicals. Apparently, the high heat of grilling reacts with proteins in red meat, poultry and fish, producing heterocyclic amines, which are linked to cancer. Another form of cancer-causing agents, polycyclic aromatic hydrocarbons, are created when juices from meats drip and hit the heat source. They then rise in smoke and can stick to the meat.

The Institute took particular aim at processed meats, such as hot dogs, sausages, bacon, ham, pastrami, salami and any meat that has been salted, smoked or cured. The chemicals used to preserve meat increase the production of cancer-causing compounds, regardless of how the meat is cooked.

The Institute's report said it "could find no amount of processed meat that is safe to eat."

High intake of fructose and sucrose: Consumption of these sugars may increase the risk of developing pancreatic cancer, according to a new study conducted by researchers from the University of Hawaii and the University of Southern California. Fructose naturally occurs in fruits, while sucrose is usually extracted from sugar cane or sugar beets. Researchers analyzed dietary data on 162,150 people who had participated in the Hawaii-Los Angeles Multiethnic Cohort Study, looking for evidence that a diet with a high glycemic load increases the risk of pancreatic cancer. Participants who ate the most fructose had a significantly higher pancreatic cancer risk than those who consumed the least. Participants who drank more fruit juice also had a higher risk of pancreatic cancer. Meanwhile, among obese and overweight patients, high sucrose intake was correlated with a higher risk of pancreatic cancer.

Smoking cigarettes: This increases the incidence of any type of cancer by undermining the blood's ability to carry oxygen to the cells of the body and inflaming them. In additon, smoking and second-hand smoke cause cadmium poisoning, a major risk for developing cancer.

Sunscreens: Cancer of all types increased dramatically when sunscreens and sunglasses were introduced to the masses. (See Chapter 4 for details.)

Night shift work: The World Health Organization's International Agency for Research on Cancer (IARC) has added working the night shift to a list of possible carcinogens, based on an analysis of the existing research on the topic. The IARC reviewed studies on night workers, primarily nurses and airline crews, and found night workers were more likely to develop cancer than day workers. "There was enough of a pattern in people who do shift work to recognize that there's an increase in cancer," said IARC carcinogen classifications unit head Vincent Cogliano. Apparently, years of overnight work among women is particularly linked to higher breast cancer, with a similar effect on prostate cancer in men.

Blood transfusions: If you opt for cancer surgery and receive a blood transfusion, please be aware that this may significantly increase your risk of heart attack and death. New research shows that blood transfusions increase the risk of complications and reduce survival rates. Almost immediately after it is donated, blood begins to lose its ability to transport oxygen to the cells of the patient's body. The longer the blood has been stored, the higher the risk of heart attack, heart failure, stroke and death.

Nitric oxide in red blood cells is critical to the delivery of oxygen to the body's tissues. If blood is stored for more than two weeks, its nitric oxide concentration drops to a level that may endanger the life of the patient. Current practice is to store blood for transfusion for up to six weeks. The above risk could be reduced by enriching the blood with nitric oxide, but very few hospitals do so.

In a study reported in the March 20, 2008 *New England Journal of Medicine*, researchers found that patients who were given older units of blood had higher rates of in-hospital mortality. At one year, mortality was significantly less in the patients given newer blood. In another study, at the University of Bristol, researchers found that patients receiving a red blood cell transfusion were three times more likely to experience complications from lack of oxygen to key organs, such as heart attack or stroke. And an earlier study at Duke University in 2004 found that patients who receive a blood transfusion to treat blood loss or anemia were twice as likely to die during their first 30 days of hospitalization. They were also more than three times as likely to suffer a heart attack within 30 days, when compared to those who did not receive a transfusion.

Note: There are alternative options to blood transfusion that carry a much lower risk, such as auto-transfusion and hemodilution (for details, see *Timeless Secrets of Health and Rejuvenation).*

Ionizing radiation: Exposure can increase the risk of certain cancers. **X-rays** used to treat disorders such as acne or adenoid enlargement can increase the risk of certain types of leukemia and lymphoma. Your doctor will not tell you this, but x-rays accumulate in the body, and each x-ray taken increases the risk, regardless whether it has been given for your teeth, gallbladder, spine, lungs, or bones.

In 2006, over 62 million **CT** or **Cat** scans were performed in the United States, which has greatly increased the personal radiation dose experienced by the average U.S. resident. The radiation dose from a CT scan is 50 to 100 times larger than from a conventional x-ray. A surge in the use of CT scans in the last 25 years has led to millions of patients per year being unnecessarily exposed to dangerous radiation that increases their risk of cancer, according to a paper published in the *New England Journal of Medicine*.

There are no harmless **MRIs** or **mammograms**. Other studies reveal that children exposed to x-rays are more likely to develop breast cancer as adults. Microwave ovens that heat and radiate your food are just as damaging and can cause cancer of the blood, as well as tumors in the brain and other parts of the body. (See section below.)

Facts about mammography:

- Each x-ray you are exposed to increases your risk of abnormal cell growth. One standard mammography test results in approximately 1 rad (radiation absorbed dose) exposure, about 1,000 times greater than that from a chest x-ray.
- The National Cancer Institute (NCI) reports that among women under 35, mammography could cause 75 cases of breast cancer for every 15 it identifies.
- A Canadian study found a 52 percent increase in breast cancer mortality in young women who have received annual mammograms.
- Dr. Charles B. Simone, a former clinical associate in immunology and pharmacology at the National Cancer Institute, said, "Mammograms increase the risk for developing breast cancer and raise the risk of spreading or metastasizing an existing growth."
- After reviewing 117 studies conducted between 1966 and 2005, an expert panel from the American College of Physicians (ACP) found the data on mammography screening for women in their 40s are so unclear that the effectiveness of reducing breast cancer death could be either 15% or " ... nearly zero."

167

- Researchers at the Nordic Cochrane Centre in Denmark found that for every 2,000 women who received mammograms over a 10-year period, only <u>one</u> would have her life prolonged, but 10 would endure unnecessary and potentially harmful treatments. The study examined the benefits and negative effects of seven breast cancer screening programs on 500,000 women in the United States, Canada, Scotland and Sweden.
- Dr. Samuel Epstein of the Cancer Prevention Coalition claims, "Screening mammography poses significant and cumulative risks of breast cancer for pre-menopausal women." ..."The premenopausal breast is highly sensitive to radiation, each 1 rad exposure increasing breast cancer risk by about 1 percent, with a cumulative 10 percent increased risk for each breast over a decade's screening," says Dr. Samuel Epstein, one of the top cancer experts in the world.
- The strong compression of breasts during the mammography procedure may help disperse existing cancer cells. Medical schools teach doctors to always handle woman's breasts with great care for this reason.
- Research has identified a gene, called oncogene AC, that is extremely sensitive to even small doses of radiation. A significant percentage of women in the United States have this gene, which could increase their risk of mammography-induced cancer. An estimated 10,000 AC carriers will die of breast cancer each year due to mammography.
- Since mammogram screening was introduced, the incidence of a form of breast cancer called ductal carcinoma in situ (DCIS) has increased by 328%.
- Each year, thousands of women unnecessarily undergo mastectomies, radiation and chemotherapy after receiving false positives on a mammogram.
- In July 1995, *The Lancet* wrote about mammograms, saying "The benefit is marginal, the harm caused is substantial, and the costs incurred are enormous ..."

As published in October 2007 by *The Cochrane Library and PubMed* (October 2007), self-breast exams don't benefit mortality rates from breast cancer either. Two large population-based studies (388,535 women) from Russia and Shanghai that compared breast self-examination found that death rates from breast cancer were the same among women who rigorously self-examined as those who did not. Almost twice as many biopsies (3,406) with benign results were performed in the screening groups compared to the control groups (1,856).

Dr. Epstein, who is also a professor emeritus of Environmental and Occupational Medicine at the University of Illinois School of Public Health, has been warning about the risks of mammography since at least 1992. Commenting on the official mammography guidelines, Epstein says: "They were conscious, chosen, politically expedient acts by a small group of people for the sake of their own power, prestige and financial gain, resulting in suffering and death for millions of women. They fit the classification of **crimes against humanity**."

Experts now no longer recommend following a strict examination routine, but rather for women to get to know what is normal, and feel their breasts regularly for signs of any changes. They should look out for a new lump or hard knot found in the breast or armpit, or unusual changes in the size, color, shape or symmetry of the breast and nipple, such as swelling or thickening of the breast.

Is there a good alternative screening method?

Yes, there is a side-effect free and inexpensive screening technology that is far more effective than mammography. High-resolution Digital Infrared Thermal Imaging (DITI). DITI measures the radiation of infrared heat from your body and translates this information into anatomical images. If there is an abnormal growth of some sort in your breast, it will stand out clearly on the thermographic image as a "hot spot."

Although accepted by Duke University, this diagnostic tool is not a mainstream technology. "...The establishment ignores safe and effective alternatives to mammography, particularly trans illumination with infrared scanning," Dr. Epstein points out.

Thanks to the discoveries of the North Carolina Institute of Technology (NCIT), a privately funded research center, thermal imaging, done using the protocol established by NCIT, may find developing breast cancer 10 years earlier than mammography. (Check out BreastCancerCured.com for more information.)

Comment: I personally don't endorse any screening method to diagnose cancer, for reasons explained in this book. Just having the fear and expectation that you may have breast cancer, when you really do not, focuses your mind on disease, which is often enough to actually trigger an illness in your body. In addition, the pressure that doctors and loved ones may put on you to get the "proper treatment" can be so overwhelming that you feel you have no other choice but to go ahead with it. Feeling trapped or cornered while feeling physically ill is certainly not conducive for healing to occur. It is by far more beneficial to attend to the underlying causes of congestion in the body, as outlined in this book, than to treat the symptoms of the lymph congestion behind abnormal changes of the breast. The same principle holds true for every so-called disease.

Chapter Six

What You Need to Know
to Heal Yourself

Cancer—Who Cures It?

Those who have gone into complete remission of cancer and remained free from it are the most likely candidates to reveal the mechanisms that cause and cure cancer.

Anne was 43 when she was diagnosed with an incurable form of lymphoma and was given only a short time to live. Her doctors strongly recommended that she have radiation and chemotherapy treatments, the two most commonly used methods of combating cancer cells. Anne was aware that the treatments could not only substantially increase the risk of secondary cancer, but also have potentially severe side effects. She refused the treatment, arguing that if the cancer was incurable anyway, why treat it and unnecessarily suffer the horrendous side effects.

Having accepted that she had an incurable disease, which meant that she had come to terms with death, Anne felt free to look for alternative ways to make the "transition" easier. Rather than passively accepting her fate, she decided to focus on feeling well and began taking an *active* role in improving her wellbeing. She tried everything from acupuncture, cleansing of her organs, and herbal medicine to meditation and visualization, which were all definite signals of *caring attention* sent to her body's cells. Anne's cancer went into remission a few months later. Within a year all apparent signs of cancer had disappeared, much to the astonishment of her oncologist. Now, over two decades later, she is not only without a trace of cancer, but she also feels that she has never been healthier and more vital.

Linda was diagnosed with a malignant melanoma (the most

aggressive form of skin cancer) when she was just 38 years old. After several unsuccessful operations, she was informed that her cancer had progressed to the point that it was "terminal" and that she had only about one year to live. Linda also refused treatment with chemotherapy and radiation and, instead, focused on the more positive approaches to healing, including yoga, prayer, a vegetarian diet, cleansing her organs, meditation, and daily visualizations. Today, 22 years after having outlived her death sentence, she is as healthy as she can be with no trace of even a skin irritation.

Both Anne and Linda have changed their entire attitude toward life, from being passive victims of an uncontrollable, "invasive" disease, to being active participants in the creation of a healthy body and mind. Taking self-responsibility was their first step to remove the focus from cancer and direct it toward consciously creating healthfulness.

To call remissions such as these "miracle cures" is certainly not appropriate. Today there is ample documentation of remarkable recoveries from every type of cancer and nearly every other disorder, from diabetes to warts and even to AIDS. The fact that a spontaneous remission of cancer can occur even in the final stages of the illness, shows that the immune system not only has the potential to quickly and effectively clear the body of existing tumors, but also to prevent new ones from forming, provided their causes are addressed. A shift in attitude from "having" to attack and kill cancer cells, to leaving them in peace and eliminating the energy-depleting influences in one's life, may be a strong enough stimulant for the immune system to do away with the symptom (the cancerous tumor). Without its root causes, cancer is as harmless as a simple cold.

People like Anne and Linda do not have to be the exception; they can be the rule. So-called spontaneous remissions rarely occur spontaneously or for no apparent reason. The body regards the causes of cancer as emotional and physical obstructions that can be overcome through a healing crisis and cleansing the body as well as the mind and spirit. Active participation in the healing process and taking self-responsibility (an expression of love for oneself) is an absolute necessity in the treatment of every major disorder, including cancer. If you are afflicted with cancer, it in no way means that you are helpless.

When George, the Cypriot businessperson, came to me with kidney cancer, he was in the weakest condition of his entire life. Despite his hopeless diagnosis, George was still breathing. As long as one breathes, there is a chance of recovery. George not only recovered, but started to live his life afresh, with more awareness, love, and joy.

Cancer has the tremendous potential of creating deeper meaning and purpose in a person's life, while bringing up and releasing longstanding fears of survival and death. It can transform a pessimistic outlook on life into an optimistic one that allows the person facing cancer to perceive the positive reason behind it and everything else that happens to him in life. This inner transformation no longer allows for perceiving oneself as a helpless victim at the mercy of oncologists or surgeons. Healing cancer or a similar life-threatening condition is perhaps one of the most powerful and meaningful accomplishments a person can achieve in life.

Removing the Need for Cancer

Having examined a great number of cancer patients in my European practice during the 1990s, I discovered that all of them, regardless of the type of cancer, had accumulated large quantities of gallstones in the liver and gallbladder. By removing *all* stones from the liver and gallbladder through a series of liver cleanses, and cleansing the colon and kidneys before and after each liver flush[44], a person creates the physical preconditions for most every type of cancer to go into spontaneous remission. This also applies to cancers that are commonly considered terminal.

If the health-seeker hence forward maintains a healthy diet and lifestyle, the cure is likely to be permanent. Evidence abounds

---

[44] See directions for these cleanses in *The Amazing Liver and Gallbladder Flush.*

that plenty of fruits and vegetables have cancer-curing and cancer-preventive properties. Research carried out at Britain's Institute of Food Research has revealed that brassica vegetables such as cabbage, kale, broccoli, and Brussels sprouts contain anticarcinogenic compounds, which prompt or stimulate cancer cells to commit suicide. These vegetables have strong purifying effects on the tissues and blood. Eating them regularly greatly reduces overall toxicity and eliminates the body's need for cancer cells.

In addition to these foods, numerous herbs and plants have powerful cleansing and anticancer properties. Out of 2,500,000 plants tested, roughly 3,000 have proven anti-cancer properties. The mechanisms by which they achieve their effects vary. Some arrest the fermentation process upon which the cancer cells depend for survival (using lactic acid, for example, to generate cellular energy); others have direct toxic effects on tumor cells; still others inhibit the division of cancer cells while permitting healthy cells to reproduce normally; and finally, some affect the pH (acid/alkaline milieu) in such a way as to reduce or prevent the risks of cancer cells growing in other parts of the body. Usually, though, most of these plants have all of the above effects. A few of these are listed below.

Agaricus Blasai Mushroom (www.waiora.com/500062)
Aloe vera
Astragalus
Basil
Black cohosh** (for breast cancer)
Black walnut hull
Burdock root
Cat's claw
Cardamon
Chaparral
Coconut oil
Cogumelo do Sol (Mushrooms of the Sun)[2]
Cumin, black (nigella sativa)[45]

---

[45] Researchers at Thomas Jefferson University in Philadelphia have discovered

Dill
Ellagic acid
Essiac herbs
Fennel
Ginger*
Herbal cancer treatment Carctol (Ayurvedic herbs)
Ginseng[46]
Goji juice
Grape seed
Graviola (See section below.)
Green tea[47]
Lingzhi mushroom[48]
Licorice root (powder)[49]
Marjoram
Oregano (also oregano oil)
Parsley
Pau D 'Arco
Red clover
Rosemary

---

that an extract of nigella sativa seed oil, known as thymoquinone, can remedy one of the most virulent and difficult to treat cancers: pancreatic cancer. The extract does this by blocking pancreatic cell growth, and actually enhancing the built-in cellular function that causes programmed cell death, or apoptosis.

[46] Ginseng can increase cell oxygenation by 25%, which is very beneficial for any type of cancer.

[47] Recent studies have shown a significant preventive effect against colorectal and oral cancer in women who drank green tea regularly; and a 48% reduction in risk of developing advanced prostate cancer in men who drank five or more cups a day (over 14 years).

[48] Japan's National Cancer Center subjected this mushroom to pharmacological testing; they found that it was actually a potent immune-system builder and cancer fighter. Scientists at Japan's University School of Medicine tested the mushrooms on mice. They discovered that it retarded tumor growth by 85 percent after 20 days. Cancerous guinea pigs experienced recovery rates of over 99 percent. Lingzhi can be found for sale in many Asian markets as well as Western health shops. Extracts of "lingzhi," which may also be called "reishi," are also available.

[49] Licorice root powder is a powerful curative herb for both cancer and diabetes. It is more effective than chemotherapy drugs in destroying cancer cells, yet without injuring or destroying healthy cells.

Sage
Schizandra berry
Shiitake or Maitake mushrooms
Tumeric
Andreas Moritz kidney tea (www.presentmoment.com)
Andreas Moritz liver tea (www.presentmoment.com)
Or call +1(800) 378-3245 +1(612) 824-3157 (USA)

*Example 1:

- Ginger natural inhibits COX-2—an enzyme responsible for inflammation and pain. [*Food Chem Toxicology* 40: 1091-97,2002]
- Ginger's active ingredient, gingerol, inhibits the spread of cancer cells and makes it impossible to distinguish cancer cells from normal healthy cells. [*Cancer* Research 61: 850-53, 2001]
- Gingerol blocks inflammation and thins the blood much like aspirin does, except without the harmful side-effects that result from the use of aspirin. [*Pharmazie* 60: 83-96, 2005]
- Ginger juice produces better recovery from symptoms of nausea than ondansetron, a commonly prescribed drug during chemotherapy. [*Journal Ethnopharmacology* 62: 49-55, 1998]
- Ginger has been shown to inhibit the growth of tumors in the colon in animal studies. [*Clin Chim Acta* 358: 60-67, 2005]
- Ginger root extract (gingerols) inhibits the growth of Helicobacter pylori in the digestive tract, which is a bacterium linked to stomach cancer. [*Anticancer Research* 23: 3699-702, 2003]

**Example 2:

A French study published in the journal *Phytomedicine* showed that extract of black cohosh may prevent and halt the growth of breast cancer cells. The study was funded by the National Institutes of Health and the Susan G. Komen Breast Cancer Foundation. Black cohosh has already earned a reputation for helping with gynecological problems, kidney problems and sore throat, and relieving the symptoms of menopause. (Contraindications: Don't use black cohosh if you also use either of the two chemotherapy drugs, doxorubicin and docetaxel, or if you are pregnant).

Herbs and food substances that help heal cancer always have strong blood and tissue-cleansing effects.[50] This increases cell oxygenation, which is a prerequisite for removing the need for cancer.

In this context, Dr. Warburg's insights about the sugar-cravings of cancer cells are very helpful. Cancer cells are unable to multiply rapidly without sugar. If you have cancer, it is important that you stop eating refined, processed sugar immediately. Nutritionally, refined sugars contain none of the nutrients necessary for the assimilation of the sugar that is ingested. The eating of these sugars drains the body's stores of nutrients and energy (if any are still present), leaving less (or none) for other tasks. Cancer never kills a person; the wasting of organ tissues does. Cancer and wasting go hand in hand. Eating sugar feeds cancer cells while it starves healthy cells.

Natural sweeteners like stevia and Xylitol do not rob the body of its nutrient and energy resources. Stevia has zero calories, so it cannot serve as food for cancer cells. Xylitol contains calories (about 40% less than sugar), but its slow release into the blood gives it a much lower glycemic index. If taken in moderation, Xylitol is unlikely to pose a problem. However, refined carbohydrates, such as pasta, white bread, pastries, and cakes are quickly broken down into glucose and act just as refined sugar does. (Note: complex carbohydrates, as found in whole grains and washed white Basmati rice, are fine, but avoid most other types of polished white rice due their depleted nutritional value.) Obviously, sugar-rich foods and beverages, such as chocolate, ice cream, and soda should be avoided. The lymph-congesting dairy products like milk, yogurt, and cheese also have no place in the diet of someone seeking to recover from cancer. (Unsalted butter

---

[50] For detailed information about the healing properties of these and other common foods, spices, and herbs, see *Timeless Secrets of Health and Rejuvenation*.

is fine.) Cancer cells thrive on milk sugar (lactose).

Apart from diet and herbs, the following approaches or methods of healing may be very useful for healing the causes of cancer:

- Massage
- Art therapy
- Music therapy
- Dance therapy
- Yoga
- Physical exercise, ideally in natural light
- Regular exposure to sunlight, without using sunscreens
- Hypnosis
- Biofeedback

Sunlight—Nature's Cancer Treatment

According to a study published in the prominent *Cancer Journal* (March 2002; 94:1867-75), insufficient exposure to ultraviolet radiation may be an important risk factor for cancer in Western Europe and North America. The findings, covering mortality rates from cancer in North America, directly contradict official advice about sunlight. The research showed that deaths from a range of cancers of the reproductive and digestive systems were approximately twice as high in New England as in the Southwest, despite a diet that varies little between regions.

An examination of 506 regions found a close inverse correlation between cancer mortality and levels of UVB light. The likeliest mechanism proposed by scientists for a protective effect of sunlight is vitamin D, which is synthesized by the body when exposed to ultraviolet B rays. According to the study's author, Dr. William Grant, the northern parts of the United States may be dark enough during the winter months that vitamin D synthesis shuts down completely.

While the study focused mainly on white Americans, the researchers found that the same geographical trend affects black or dark-skinned Americans, whose overall cancer rates are significantly higher. As explained earlier, dark-skinned people require more sunlight to synthesize vitamin D.

The same study showed at least 13 malignancies are affected by a lack of sunlight, mostly reproductive and digestive cancers. The strongest inverse correlation is with breast, colon, and ovarian cancer, followed by tumors of the bladder, uterus, esophagus, rectum, and stomach.

To obtain the disease-curbing benefits of sunlight, you need to be outside at least three times a week for a minimum of 15-20 minutes. **Avoid using sunscreens and sunglasses; otherwise you won't gain the benefits from sunlight exposure. (See Chapter 4 for details.)**

[To learn about the healing powers of the sun in much more detail, and specifically, how UV-light actually prevents and cures skin cancer and why most skin cancers are caused by sun protection creams and lotions, see Chapter Eight of my book, *Timeless Secrets of Health and Rejuvenation*.]

Sleeping Enough Hours

Research shows that the immune system needs 8-9 hours of sleep in *total* darkness to recharge completely. A weak immune system cannot keep your body clean inside, and the resulting congestion threatens cellular life.

The recurring alteration of day and night regulates our natural sleep/wake cycles and essential biochemical processes. The onset of daylight triggers the release of powerful hormones (glucocorticoids), of which the main ones are cortisol and corticosterone. Their secretion has a marked circadian variation. These hormones regulate some of the most important functions in the body, including metabolism, blood sugar level, and immune responses. Peak levels occur between 4 a.m. and 8 a.m. and gradually decrease as the day continues. The lowest level occurs between midnight and 3 a.m.

By altering your natural daily sleep/wake schedule, the peak of cortisol's cycle changes as well. For example, if you continually go to sleep after midnight, instead of before 10 p.m., and/or you arise in the morning after 8 a.m. or 9 a.m., instead of with or before sunrise between 6 a.m. to 7 a.m., you will enforce a hormonal time shift (continual jet lag) that can lead to chaotic conditions in the body. Waste materials that tend to accumulate in the rectum and urinary bladder during the night are normally eliminated between 6 a.m. and 8 a.m. With a changed waking/sleeping cycle, the body has no other choice but to hold on to that waste matter and possibly reabsorb a part of it. When you disrupt your natural sleep/wake cycles, the body's biological rhythms desynchronize with the larger circadian rhythms that are controlled by the daily periods of darkness and light. This can lead to numerous types of disorders, including chronic liver disease, respiratory ailments, heart trouble, and cancer.

One of the pineal gland's most powerful hormones is the neurotransmitter *melatonin*. The secretion of melatonin starts between 9:30 and 10:30 p.m. (depending on age), inducing sleepiness. It reaches peak levels between 1 a.m. and 2 a.m. and drops to its lowest levels at midday. The pineal gland controls reproduction, sleep and motor activity, blood pressure, the immune system, the pituitary and thyroid glands, cellular growth, body temperature, and many other vital functions. All of these depend on a balanced melatonin cycle. By going to sleep late (past 10 p.m.) or working the night shift, you throw this and many other hormonal cycles out of balance.

The ongoing Nurses' Study has shown that nurses working the night shift have a more than 50% higher risk of developing cancer, but have among the lowest levels of melatonin in the blood. Higher levels of melatonin are linked with a lower risk of cancer. Blind women, for example, whose melatonin levels are naturally high (melatonin responds to darkness), have a 36 percent lower risk of breast cancer compared to sighted women. Taking a melatonin supplement has no cancer-preventing benefits, but may increase the risk because it inhibits the body's own melatonin secretion.

If you have cancer or don't want to develop it, this is about the most important advice you can get: **Get a full night's rest every night** (with the occasional exception), **beginning at no later than 10 p.m.!**

The conveniences provided by the onset of electrical lighting came with the great risk of ruining the health of millions of people. The human body and all the other organisms on the planet evolved to adjust themselves to predictable patterns of light and darkness, in a physiological cycle known as the circadian rhythm. The irregular lifestyle of modern living bypasses or ignores the body's vital need to be in synch with the daily, monthly and yearly changes of the environment. A part of your brain called the Suprachiasmatic Nucleus (SCN) controls your biological clock by closely monitoring the light and dark signals of your environment. Thus, light and darkness have the most powerful influence on our hormonal system and, in turn, on the health and vitality of every cell in the body.

When your eyes stop seeing light as it is getting dark outside, your pineal gland will begin to produce melatonin, but stops secretion altogether when you switch on a light or watch television. As a result, the sleep-inducing effect of melatonin becomes inhibited, and you may not feel sleepy at all for several more hours. In fact, the stimulation from the light at this time of the night may actually prevent you from falling asleep and cause you to develop a permanent sleeping disorder. Sleep deprivation is a common condition that afflicts 47 million American adults. And as new research indicates, it is so serious that it greatly raises their risk of cancer.

Among many other functions, melatonin triggers a nocturnal reduction in your body's estrogen levels, which significantly lowers its ability to ward off or heal **estrogen-related cancers.** By exposing yourself to nighttime light, your melatonin levels drop while your estrogen levels rise.[51] Medical scientists could not believe it at first when they learned that natural hormones such as estrogen and insulin could actually be carcinogens, but it is now official. In December 2002 the National Institute of Environmental Health Sciences (NIEHS) added estrogen to its list of known cancer-causing agents. Strong epidemiological evidence associates the hormone to breast, endometrial, and uterine cancers.

---

[51] Both men and women produce estrogen hormones.

The liver regulates numerous hormones, including estrogens and progesterone. A woman with unbalanced hormone levels[52] may experience a low sex drive (low libido), cardiovascular disease, menopausal symptoms, menstrual discomforts, PMS, breast cysts, breast cancer, fibroids, endometriosis, emotional problems, female anxiety, nervous disorders, skin problems, hair loss, and bone disorders. But it's certainly not the liver's fault when hormonal imbalance occurs. If you deprive yourself of sleep, especially the two hours before midnight, you also prevent the liver from doing its vital jobs, 500 of them.

There is no part of the body that doesn't suffer when liver functions are affected by not going to sleep on time, including the liver itself. For example, the liver removes insulin from the bloodstream, but when you interfere with its nocturnal activities (by not sleeping on time), insulin causes fat to be deposited in the liver which prevents the liver from removing insulin from the bloodstream. Elevated insulin levels lead to heart attacks, abdominal obesity, diabetes, and cancer.

Apart from making melatonin, the brain also synthesizes *serotonin* which is a very important neurotransmitter (hormone) related to our state of physical and emotional wellbeing. It affects day and night rhythms, sexual behavior, memory, appetite, impulsiveness, fear, and even suicidal tendencies. Unlike melatonin, serotonin increases with the light of day; physical exercise and sugar also stimulate it. If you get up late in the morning, the resulting lack of exposure to sufficient amounts of daylight reduces your serotonin levels throughout the day. Moreover, since melatonin is a breakdown product of serotonin, this lowers your levels of melatonin during the night. Any deviation from the circadian rhythms causes abnormal secretions of these important brain hormones. This, in turn, leads to disturbed biological rhythms, which can upset the harmonious functioning of the entire organism, including digestion, metabolism, and endocrine balance. Suddenly, you may feel "out of synch" and become susceptible to a wide variety of disorders,

---

[52] The underlying imbalance consists of a relative excess of estrogen and an absolute deficiency in progesterone.

ranging from a simple headache, bloating, and indigestion to depression and a fully grown tumor.

Note: Over 90% of serotonin is produced in the digestive system, with peak levels at noontime when the sun at its highest position. Lack of exposure to natural light or sleeping the during daytime can lead to severe gastrointestinal problems, thus affecting the health of every cell in the body.

The production of growth hormones, which stimulates growth in children and helps to maintain healthy muscle and connective tissue in adults, depends on proper sleeping cycles. Sleep triggers growth hormone production. Peak secretion occurs around 11 p.m., provided you go to sleep before 10 p.m. This short period coincides with dreamless sleep, often referred to as "beauty sleep." It is during this period of the sleep cycle that the body cleanses itself and does its main repair and rejuvenation work. If you are sleep-deprived, growth hormone production drops dramatically. To cure cancer, the body must be able to produce sufficient growth hormones. Getting enough sleep at the right time of the night is one of the best cancer-preventing and cancer-curing approaches. Moreover, it will cost you nothing and benefit you in many other ways. [For a detailed description of the body's biological rhythms and an ideal daily routine, see *Timeless Secrets of Health and Rejuvenation.*]

Maintaining Regular Meal Times

The body is controlled by numerous circadian rhythms, which regulate its most important functions in accordance with pre-programmed time intervals. Sleep, secretion of hormones and digestive juices, elimination of waste, and many other bodily processes all follow a specific daily routine. If these cyclic activities become disrupted more often than they are adhered to, the body becomes imbalanced and cannot fulfill its essential tasks. All physical activities in the body are naturally aligned with and depend on the schedule dictated by the circadian rhythms.

Having regular meal times makes it easy for the body to

prepare for the production and secretion of the right amounts of digestive juices for each meal. Irregular eating habits, on the other hand, confuse the body. Furthermore, its digestive power becomes depleted by having to adjust to a different schedule each time you eat. Skipping meals here and there, eating at different times, or eating between meals especially disrupts the cycles of bile production by the liver cells. The result is the formation of gallstones.

By maintaining a regular eating routine, the body's 60-100 trillion cells are able to receive their daily ratio of nutrients according to schedule, which helps cell metabolism to be smooth and effective. Many metabolic disorders, such as diabetes or obesity, result from irregular eating habits and can be greatly improved by matching eating times with the natural circadian rhythms.

It is best to take the largest meal of the day around midday and only light meals at breakfast (no later than 8 a.m.) and dinner (no later than 7 p.m.). Eating the main meal of the day in the evening when the digestion of food is naturally weak, leads to an overload of the gastrointestinal tract with undigested, fermenting, and putrefying food. The bacteria engaged in decomposing the undigested food produce poisons that not only affect intestinal health, but also are the main cause for developing lymphatic congestion. This causes unhealthy weight gain and disturbs basic metabolism. Cancer is a metabolic disorder that can originate in regularly eating the main meal at night and eating between meals or before going to sleep.

Overeating usually leads to intestinal congestion, the proliferation of destructive bacteria and yeast, as well as cravings for "energizing, " which really means energy-depleting, foods and beverages, such as sugar, sweets, white flour products, potato chips, chocolate, coffee, tea, and soft drinks. Constant cravings for any of these foods or beverages indicate cellular starvation. Such starvation at the cellular level may force the weakest cells in the body to undergo genetic mutation.

Eating a Vegan-Vegetarian Diet

Vegetarians have believed all along that living on a purely vegetarian diet can improve health and the quality of life. More recently, medical research has found that a properly balanced vegetarian diet may in fact be the healthiest diet. This was demonstrated by the over 11,000 volunteers who participated in the *Oxford Vegetarian Study* which for a period of 15 years analyzed the effects of a vegetarian diet on longevity, heart disease, cancer, and various other diseases.

The results of the study stunned the vegetarian community as much as the meat-producing industry: "Meat eaters are twice as likely to die from heart disease, have a 60 percent greater risk of dying from cancer and a 30 percent higher risk of death from other causes." In addition, the incidence of obesity, which is a major risk factor in many diseases, including cancer, gallbladder disease, hypertension, and adult onset diabetes, was found to be much lower in those following a vegetarian diet. In a study of 50,000 vegetarians, the American National Institute of Health found that vegetarians live longer and have an impressively lower incidence of heart disease. They also have significantly lower rates of cancer than meat-eating Americans have.

What we eat has a critical impact on our health. According to the American Cancer Society, up to 35% of the nearly 900,000 new cases of cancer each year in the United States could be prevented by following proper dietary recommendations. Researcher Rollo Russell writes in his *Notes on the Causation of Cancer:* "I have found of twenty five nations eating flesh largely, nineteen had a high cancer rate and only one had a low rate, and that of thirty five nations eating little or no flesh, none of these had a high rate." Furthermore, T. Colin Campbell, Ph.D. and Thomas M. Campbell, authors of *The China Study*, succinctly sum up the results of their groundbreaking research in the field of nutrition science: "The people who eat the most animal protein have the most heart disease, cancer and diabetes." Not surprisingly, they recommend a whole foods, plant-based diet. Their research indicates that "the lower the percentage of animal-based foods that are consumed, the greater the health benefits—even when that percentage declines for 10% to 0% of calories. So it's not unreasonable to assume that the optimum percentage of animal-based products is zero, at least for anyone with a predisposition for a degenerative disease."

Could cancer lose its grip on modern societies if they turned to a balanced vegetarian diet? The answer is "yes" according to two major reports, one by the World Cancer Research Fund and the other by the Committee on the Medical Aspects of Food and Nutrition Policy in the UK. The reports conclude that a diet rich in plant foods and the maintenance of a healthy body weight could prevent four million cases of cancer worldwide. Both reports stress the need for increasing one's intake of plant fiber, fruits, and vegetables and reducing red and processed meat consumption to less than 80-90g per day.

Eating a balanced vegetarian diet is one of the most effective ways to prevent cancer. If you feel you cannot solely live on foods that are of vegetable origin, then at least try to substitute chicken, rabbit, or turkey for red meat for a period of time. Eventually, you may feel confident enough to eat a fully vegetarian diet. All forms of animal protein decrease the solubility of bile, which is a major risk factor for developing gallstones, as well as lymph and blood vessel wall congestion. These are the main causes of cell mutation, which lead to cancer.

[For complete guidelines on how to eat a healthy, life-sustaining diet according to your body type's unique requirements, see *Timeless Secrets of Health and Rejuvenation*.]

Exercise and Cancer

Is exercise beneficial to cancer patients or is it harmful? New research clears up any controversy and points to the benefits of exercise as a means of fighting cancer, according to a 2007 online-report issued by Johns Hopkins University. For cancer patients undergoing chemotherapy, exercise is one of the best ways to combat treatment-related fatigue. "It's not recommended that you begin an intense, new exercise regimen while undergoing chemotherapy, but if you exercised before your cancer diagnosis, try and maintain some level of activity," says Deborah Armstrong, M.D., Associate Professor of Oncology, Gynecology, and Obstetrics at Johns Hopkins. "If you haven't been exercising, try low-level exercise, such as walking or swimming."

The benefits of exercise are not limited to helping treatment-related fatigue. In fact, they actively contribute to curing cancer. Several groundbreaking studies attest to this fact. This hardly comes as a surprise, since cancer cells are typically oxygen-deprived, and exercise is a direct way to deliver extra oxygen to cells throughout the body and to improve the immune response. Researchers also believe that exercise can regulate the production of certain hormones that, unregulated, may spur tumor growth.

Exercise should not be strenuous, however. Exercising for half an hour each day or several hours a week may be all that is needed to significantly increase cell oxygenation. (Please refer to Chapter six of my book, *Timeless Secrets of Health and Rejuvenation*, for proper guidance on healthy exercising programs suitable for specific body types, and breathing exercises that greatly enhance oxygenation of cells.)

In one study, published in the *Journal of the American Medical Association*, researchers followed 2,987 women with breast cancer. Women who, for example, walked more than one hour a week after their cancer diagnosis were less likely to die of their breast cancer. In another study of 573 women, those who followed a moderate exercise program for more than six hours a week after a colon cancer diagnosis were 61% less likely to die of cancer-specific causes than women who exercised less than one hour per week. In all cases, exercise was found to be a protective factor regardless of the patient's age, stage of cancer, or weight. A third study, published in the *Journal of Clinical Oncology*, confirmed the above findings after examining the effects of exercise on 832 men and women with stage III colon cancer.

Restoring Chi—The Life Force

"It is the life force which cures diseases because a dead man needs no more medicines." ~ Samuel Hahnemann, founder of homeopathy.

In other words, when the life force, Chi, is depleted, not even the best of medicines can restore a sick man's health or bring a dead man back to life. The life force is the only power in the body that is capable of healing it from an illness.

Ener-Chi Art is a unique method of healing art based on energized oil paintings that I created to help restore a balanced flow of Chi or vital energy through the organs and systems in the body. With any cancer, Chi-flow is severely disrupted throughout the body. When applied in the context of physical cleansing and healing, I consider this unique approach a very important and effective tool in facilitating a more successful outcome of any treatment or healing method.

When the cells of the body experience a balanced flow of Chi, they are better able to remove toxic wastes, absorb more of the oxygen, water, and nutrients they need, do necessary repair work, and increase their overall performance and vitality. Although I consider the combination of liver/colon/kidney cleanses to be one of the most effective tools to help the body return to balanced functioning, years of congestion and deterioration may hinder the body from fully restoring its Chi. My ten years of research with this method, which took me almost two years to develop, has shown that Ener-Chi Art may very well accomplish this balanced Chi flow. Its rate of effectiveness so far has been 100% for every person who has been exposed to the artwork. Due to their unique healing effects, all the Ener-Chi Art paintings were once exhibited for over a month at the prestigious *Abbott Northwestern Hospital* in Minneapolis, Minnesota for all the patients to view. Three of my original paintings—for the immune system, the lymphatic system, and blood circulation/small intestine—hung in the cancer ward, affording all cancer patients the opportunity to experience their healing properties.

Ener-Chi Art is perhaps one of the most profound and

instantly effective healing programs to balance the life force, Chi, in the following organs, parts, and systems of the body:

1. Back
2. Blood
3. Brain & nervous system
4. Ears
5. Eyes
6. Endocrine system
7. Heart
8. Immune system
9. Joints
10. Kidneys and bladder
11. Large intestine
12. Liver
13. Lymphatic system
14. Muscular system
15. Neck & shoulders
16. Nose & sinuses
17. Respiratory system
18. Small intestine & circulatory system
19. Skeletal system
20. Skin
21. Spleen
22. Stomach
23. Tongue

I have also created one painting for general health, one for transmuting emotional and physical trauma called *Beyond the Horizon*, and other paintings to balance our relationship with the water and air elements; the rocks and mountains; the animal kingdom; the plant kingdom; and the world of nature spirits. Fully energized prints for each of these paintings are available through my website.

The desired benefits occur while viewing the Ener-Chi Art paintings for about 30 seconds.[53]

---

[53] For more information on Ener-Chi Art and to order the pictures, see the

Sacred Santémony—
for Emotional Healing and More

Sacred Santémony is a unique healing system that uses sounds from specific words to balance deep emotional/spiritual imbalances. The powerful words in Sacred Santémony are produced from whole-brain use (involving both hemispheres of the brain) of the letters of the *ancient languages*—languages that are comprised of the basic sound frequencies that underlie and bring forth all physical manifestation. The letters of the ancient language vibrate at a much higher level than our modern languages, and when combined to form whole words, they generate feelings of peace and harmony (Santémony) to calm the storms of unrest, violence, and turmoil, both internal and external.

I began this system of healing in April 2002 when I spontaneously began to chant sounds in ancient languages, including Native Americans, Tibetan, Sanskrit and others. Within two weeks, I was able to bring forth sounds that would instantly remove emotional blocks and resistance or aversion to certain situations and people, foods, chemicals, thought forms, beliefs, etc. The following are a few examples of conditions Sacred Santémony has improved:

- Reducing or removing fear related to the past or future, death, disease, the body, foods, harmful chemicals, parents and other people, lack of abundance, impoverishment, phobias, and environmental threats.
- Clearing or reducing the pain from a recent or current hurt, disappointment, or anger resulting from past emotional trauma or negative experiences in life.
- Cleansing of the *Akashic Records* (a recording of all experiences the soul has gathered throughout all life streams) from persistent fearful elements, including the idea and

author's website http://www.ener-chi.com or *Other Books, Products and Services by the Author* at the end of this book.

concept that we are separate from and not one with Spirit, God, or our Higher Self.

- Setting the preconditions for the individual to resolve his/her karmic issues, not through pain and suffering, but through creativity and joy.
- Improving or clearing up allergies and intolerances to foods, gluten, chemical substances, pesticides, herbicides, air pollutants, radiation, medicinal drugs, pharmaceutical byproducts, etc.
- Alleviating the psycho-emotional root causes of chronic illness, including cancer, heart disease, MS, diabetes, arthritis, brain disorders, depression, and the like.
- Resolving other difficulties or barriers in life by converting them into the useful blessings that they really are.

Note: Please see the section *Other Books, Products, and Services by the Author* at the end of the book for further details on how to arrange for a session of Sacred Santémony with Andreas (via telephone). The benefits of Sacred Santémony become amplified when combined with the viewing of Ener-Chi Art pictures.

Graviola—More Effective Than Chemo

If you suffer from cancer and feel you need to have a specific treatment that is both natural and at least as effective as chemotherapy or radiation, you may wish to consider the use of the herbal remedy Graviola. Graviola is a plant indigenous to most of the warmest tropical areas in South and North America, including the Amazon.

Scientists have been studying Graviola's properties since the 1940s and discovered it has numerous active compounds and chemicals. Graviola has shown a large variety of benefits for many different ailments, one of which is cancer. Graviola contains a set of chemicals called *Annonaceous acetogenins*. It makes these compounds in its leaves and stem, bark, and fruit seeds. In a total of eight clinical studies, several independent research groups have confirmed that these chemicals have significant anti-tumor properties and selective toxicity against various types of cancer cells without harming healthy cells. Purdue University, in West Lafayette, Indiana, has conducted a great deal of research on these chemicals called *acetogenins*, much of which has been funded by The National Cancer Institute and/or the National Institute of Health (NIH). Thus far, Purdue University and/or its staff have filed at least nine U.S. and/or international patents for their work on the anti-tumor and insecticidal properties and uses of these acetogenins.

One of America's billion-dollar drug companies attempted to produce an anti-cancer drug from Graviola after it discovered that this compound was 10,000 times more toxic to colon cancer cells than a common chemo drug. It found Graviola to be lethal to 12 different kinds of malignant cells, especially those that cause lung, prostate, and breast cancers, and to be safe enough to protect healthy cells instead of killing them. With Graviola, the patient experiences no nausea or hair loss, and no major weight loss or weakness. Rather than compromising the immune system, Graviola actually strengthens it.

For seven years, this drug company tried to develop a synthetic patented prescription version of Graviola's anti-cancer chemicals (it being against the law to patent natural compounds), but all attempts failed and the project was terminated. Instead of making their findings public, the researchers boxed up their results and put their research away for good. Eventually, though, the story leaked out and Graviola is now increasingly receiving the recognition it deserves among health professionals and researchers alike.

Many terminal cases of cancer have been reversed through the use of Graviola, even in people 85 years or older. When cancerous tumors break up, the body may be flooded with poisons, causing the patient to feel quite weak. To minimize the intensity of the healing crisis, it is important to cleanse the colon every day, perhaps through such means as enemas, colemas, or colosan. The kidneys should be supported by drinking the kidney cleanse tea. (For this recipe see *Timeless Secrets of Health and Rejuvenation* or *The Amazing Liver and Gallbladder Flush*.) If possible, the liver should be cleansed as well.

Note: Graviola has cardio-depressant, vasodilator, and hypotensive (lowers blood pressure) actions. The dosage should be increased gradually. Overly large dosages can cause nausea and vomiting. Use this treatment only when under the supervision of a health practitioner who understands its value, the above actions, and its possible interaction with other drugs.

Miracle Mineral Supplement (MMS)

All cancers have three things in common: 1. the immune system is weak and depleted; 2. the body is overwhelmed with toxins and waste matter; 3. there is a massive presence of pathogens (infecting agents) inside and around cancer cells. These may include parasites, viruses, bacteria, yeast, and fungi. One mineral substance—sodium chlorite—may have the most balanced and immediate effects on all these disease-causing factors. Apart from the topics already discussed, other important requirements for healing cancer and most illnesses, both serious and minor, include the following:

1. Neutralize the toxins and poisons that weaken the immune system and feed or attract the pathogens.
2. Strengthen the immune system to remove all pathogens and keep them at bay.
3. While detoxifying, kill off all harmful parasites, viruses, bacteria, fungi, molds, and yeast and eliminate them from the body.

To be successful, all of these need to occur at the same time.

The product *Miracle Mineral Supplement* (MMS) is a stabilized oxygen solution of 28% sodium chlorite (not "chloride") in distilled water. When a small amount of lemon juice, lime juice or citric acid solution is added to a few drops of MMS, chlorine dioxide is formed. Once ingested, the chlorine dioxide instantly oxidizes harmful substances such as parasites, bacteria, viruses, yeast, fungi, and molds within a matter of hours, while boosting the immune system at least tenfold. By doing so, MMS has removed, for example, any strands of the malaria and HIV viruses from the blood within less than 48 hours in nearly every person tested. MMS has also been used successfully for many other serious illnesses, including Hepatitis A, B, & C, typhoid, most cancers, herpes, pneumonia, food poisoning, tuberculosis, asthma, and influenza.

The following is a quote from a book by Jim Humble, the discoverer of MMS and the author of the book, *Breakthrough . . . the Miracle Mineral Supplement of the 21st Century:*

"While first developed to address Malaria in Africa, it has now been shown to address any disease condition that is directly or indirectly related to pathogens. There is documentation of over 75,000 cases of Malaria being overcome in Africa. Often in as little as 4 hours all symptoms are gone, and the patient is tested clear of Malaria. It is now known that MMS can be used to overcome the symptoms of AIDS, Hepatitis A, B & C, Typhoid, most cancers, herpes, pneumonia, food poisoning, tuberculosis, asthma, colds, flu and a host of other conditions. Even conditions not directly related to pathogens seem to be helped due to the huge boost to the body's immune system, for example, macular degeneration, allergies, lupus, inflammatory bowel disorders, diabetes, snake bites, abscessed teeth and fibromyalgia. Please note that MMS doesn't cure anything, but rather it allows our body to heal itself. Notice how I carefully step around the words 'cure' and 'heal', even though that is what is really happening."

Humble says, "Separate tests conducted by the Malawi government produced 99% cure results for malaria. Over 60% of AIDS victims treated with MMS in Uganda were well in 3 days, with 98% well within one month. More than 90% of the malaria victims were well in 4 to 8 hours. Dozens of other diseases were successfully treated and can be controlled with this new mineral supplement."

The inventor believes that this information is too important to the world for any one person or group to control. The free e-book (digital book) download gives complete details of this discovery. Please help to ensure that it gets to the world free. Many medical breakthroughs have been suppressed, and this invention must not be added to that list. The name of the e-book is *The Miracle Mineral Supplement of the 21st Century.* You can download it free of charge or ask a friend to download and print it for you if you don't have a computer. The website address is www.miraclemineral.org. Jim Humble's book tells the story of the discovery and how to make and use it. I recommend that every person read this book. Jim has no personal, vested interest in making MMS available to the world. Rather, he wants to use his discovery to end disease and poverty. For more information and to purchase MMS, visit, or call toll free: 866.258.4006 (USA) or 709.570.7401 (Canada).

Ojibwa Herb Tea—8-Herb Essiac—
One Remedy for Many Ailments?

Ojibwa Indian herb tea is a 280-year-old Native American Indian root and herb tea remedy made in the "1700's" by the Ojibwa Indian medicine society. Ojibwa people used it to survive a smallpox genocide started by the early European settlers.

Native Americans have since used the tea formula to cure all types of cancers, type I and type II diabetes, liver infections and other liver/gallbladder conditions, tumors, arthritis, gout, asthma and other respiratory ailments, obesity, high blood pressure, elevated cholesterol, fibromyalgia and chronic fatigue syndrome, ulcers, irritable bowel syndrome (IBS), kidney and bladder disorders, sinus congestion, influenza (flu) and chest colds, measles, mumps, chicken pox, smallpox, herpes, diarrhea, constipation, lymph edema (fluid retention), heart disease, allergies, skin diseases, auto immune diseases such as lupus and AIDS, Lyme disease, addiction to substances such as alcohol, drugs, and tobacco, clinical depression, and much more.

Eight-herb Essiac contains the following ingredients:

Blessed Thistle is used for digestive problems such as gas, constipation, and an upset stomach. This herb is also used to treat liver and gallbladder diseases.
Burdock Root is a mild diuretic. It increases the production of both urine and sweat, potentially making it useful for treating

swelling and fever. Burdock root might play a role in preventing liver damage caused by alcohol, chemicals, or medications. The exact reason for this protective effect is not known, but it is thought to involve opposition to a chemical process called oxidation, which occurs in the body as a natural function of metabolism. Although oxidation is a natural process, that doesn't mean it isn't harmful to the body! One result of oxidation is the release of oxygen free radicals, which are chemicals that may suppress immune function. Antioxidants such as burdock root may protect body cells from damage caused by oxidation.

Kelp is a sea vegetable that is a concentrated source of minerals, including iodine, potassium, magnesium, calcium, and iron. Kelp as a source of iodine assists in making the thyroid hormones, which are necessary for maintaining normal metabolism in all cells of the body. This increases energy levels and makes it easier to maintain a healthy body weight. Kelp is the most nutrient-dense of all the Native Ojibwa tea ingredients—and it isn't found in the four-herb formulas of the tea.

Red Clover is a source of many valuable nutrients, including calcium, chromium, magnesium, niacin, phosphorus, potassium, thiamine, and vitamin C. Red clover is also one of the richest sources of isoflavones (water-soluble chemicals that act like estrogens and are found in many plants). The isoflavones found in red clover have been studied for their effectiveness in treating some forms of cancer. It is thought that the isoflavones prevent the proliferation of cancer cells and that they may even destroy them.

Sheep Sorrel is a rich source of oxalic acid, sodium, potassium, iron, manganese, phosphorous, beta carotene, and vitamin C. This Native Ojibwa tea ingredient is a mild diuretic, mild antiseptic, and mild laxative.

Slippery Elm Bark has been used as a poultice for cuts and bruises. It is also useful for aching joints due to gout or other causes. Besides being a Native American tea ingredient, this herb is often used to alleviate sore throats. Slippery elm bark is found in many lozenges that claim to soothe throat irritation. Since a sore throat and a cough are often linked, slippery elm bark has also been used in cough remedies. Furthermore, it regulates the

196

elimination phase of the digestive process, easing both constipation and diarrhea.

Turkish Rhubarb Root is a detoxifying herb that is world-famous for its healing properties. Rhubarb root purges the body of bile, parasites, and stagnating food in the stomach by stimulating the gall duct to expel toxic waste matter. It alleviates chronic liver problems by cleansing the liver. Rhubarb root improves digestion and helps regulate the appetite. It has also helped to heal ulcers, alleviate disorders of the spleen and colon, relieve constipation, and heal hemorrhoids and bleeding in the upper digestive tract.

Watercress is high in vitamin C, and is used as a general tonic. Its bitter taste is thought to regulate the appetite and improve digestion. It can be used to alleviate nervous conditions, constipation, and liver disorders. Watercress is a popular cough and bronchitis remedy. It contains a remarkable substance called rhein, which appears to inhibit the growth of pathogenic bacteria in the intestines. It is believed that rhein is also effective against Candida Albicans (yeast infection), fever and inflammation, and pain.

Caution: As with other sources of food and remedies that contain soluble fiber, such as slippery elm bark, Ojibwa tea can interfere with the absorption of other medicines within the gut if they are taken at the same time. Because of this, take prescription medications at an alternate time to consuming this tea.

Where to find it: One company sells this tea formula under the name Essiac tea at http://www.premium-essiac-tea-4less.com. For those who wish to purchase these herbs separately, the exact breakdown of herbs (ratio) is available at this web page: http://www.biznet1.com/p2699.htm. This site also sells the Ojibwa tea in larger quantities.

The Bicarbonate Maple Syrup Treatment

Although sugar intake strongly stimulates cancer cell growth, the combination of baking soda (sodium bicarbonate) and maple syrup has the exact opposite effect; it makes it actually very difficult for cancer cells to function and survive.

Cancer cells can only operate in an acidic and oxygen-deprived environment. Since they are anaerobic by nature, they cannot use oxygen to metabolize glucose (sugar) and produce energy, but, instead, they have to ferment it. Compared with aerobic cells, which use oxygen and glucose to produce energy, cancer cells require about 15 times the amount of glucose as healthy cells to generate the same amount of metabolic energy. The cancer cells' excessive hunger for glucose robs other healthy cells of this vital nutrient, thereby causing them to become weak, die, or also mutate into cancer cells. The starvation or weakening of healthy cells caused by the cancer cells' incessant draining of nutrients from the tissue fluids, greatly diminishes the affected organ's glucose and energy reserves. This is the main reason behind the failure of organs associated with cancer.

To prepare this simple, inexpensive but powerful remedy, combine pure 5 parts of 100% maple syrup (ideally B-grade), with 1 part of pure baking soda (with no added aluminum!).[54] Place the mixture in a sauce pan and heat it on a medium flame for five minutes. Stir briskly. The mixture will greatly spread out and become foamy. Store in a cool place and take one teaspoon twice daily. For very serious conditions, take one teaspoon three times a day. Take uninterruptedly for at least 7-8 days, which is often sufficient to collapse tumors of the size 1-2 inches. You may experience a strong die-off, consisting of dead cancer cells, bacteria, and toxins, usually expelled via the intestinal tract. Don't be concerned if diarrhea occurs. This is the body's way of relieving itself of the acid burden that's behind the cancer. Other, seemingly unrelated health conditions may improve, too.

The maple syrup is capable of transporting bicarbonate into all parts of body, including the brain and nervous system, bones, teeth, joints, eyes, and solid tumors. It may also help with other conditions of acidosis. Sodium bicarbonate therapy is harmless and so quick-acting because it is extremely diffusible.

---

[54] Bob's Red Mill or other brands state "Aluminum-free" on their labels.

The greatest advocate of sodium bicarbonate as a cancer therapy is the prominent oncologist, Dr. Tullio Simoncini in Rome, Italy. The basic concept of his therapy consists of administering a solution of sodium bicarbonate directly into tumors. He believes that cancer is a fungus which can be destroyed by direct exposure to sodium bicarbonate.

Dr. Simoncini is certainly correct about fungus playing a major role in nearly all cancers. There are over 1.5 million different species of fungus. One of them is Candida Albicans which grows in the intestinal tract to help ferment undigested sugars or starches. This intestinal yeast can spread to other parts of the body and set up colonies wherever the need for decomposing organic waste arises.

Certain fungi, in particular "'white rot" fungi, can degrade insecticides, herbicides, pentachlorophenol, creosote, coal tars, and heavy fuels and turn them into carbon dioxide, water, and basic elements. Fungi occur in every environment on Earth and play very important roles in most ecosystems, including the internal ecosystem of the body. Along with bacteria, fungi are the major decomposers in most terrestrial and some aquatic ecosystems. As decomposers, they play an indispensable role in nutrient cycling, especially as saprotrophs and symbionts, degrading organic matter to inorganic molecules. They become essential when the body accumulates organic waste matter, heavy metals and chemical compounds.[55] They will also turn up when cells decay, die, and may not be readily removed via the body's lymphatic system. Congested lymphatic ducts are almost always causing fungal proliferations in the cells and tissues of organs. The fungi that grow in the tissues of organs always show up as a white mass. That's why cancerous tumors are always white

---

[55] When compared with healthy tissues, cancer tissues contain a much higher concentration of toxic chemicals, pesticides, and heavy metals. In 1973, a study conducted by the Department of Occupational Health at Hebrew University-Hadassah Medical School in Jerusalem found a significantly higher concentration of such toxic compounds as DDT and PCB's in cancerous breast tissue of women, compared with the normal breast and adjacent adipose tissue in the same women.

(although on scanning images they show up as dark masses or shadows).

While doing their precious job, fungi produce compounds with biological activity. Several of these compounds are toxic and are therefore called mycotoxins, referring to their fungal origin and toxic activity. Particularly infamous are the aflatoxins, which are insidious liver toxins and highly carcinogenic metabolites. In other words, the fungal toxins can damage cells and cause them to mutate into cancer calls. In essence, fungi grow inside and outside polluted tissue to feed on the harmful toxins and chemicals, but they also produce poisons which can further damage cells and cause them to mutate. Thus, while the fungal activity helps remove the causes of the original cancer (toxins), the poisons the fungi produce contributes to the cancer's proliferation.

Bicarbonate of soda can bind to and remove toxins, chemicals, and organic acidic waste matter, and it quickly raises the pH of cancer cells and their environment. The extracellular pH of solid tumors is significantly more acidic compared to normal tissues. By altering the pH of a tumor it becomes exposed to more oxygen, which can cause its destruction.

To get as close as possible to the tumor tissue, Dr. Simoncini places a small catheter directly into the artery that nourishes the tumor, and administers high doses of sodium bicarbonate to the deepest recesses of the tumor. He claims that most tumors treated in this way will break up within several days, similar to the maple syrup bicarbonate treatment.

Marine Phytoplankton—
Nature's Ultimate Superfood

Marine Phytoplankton is considered to be one of the most powerful foods on Earth because it is loaded with high-energy super anti-oxidants, vitamins, minerals, and proteins in microscopic form. It is a tiny little plant (about the size of a red blood cell) that naturally grows in the ocean and is the beginning of the food chain, whereas all other living creatures in the ocean feed on other living things that feed on this little plant. It is responsible for over 70% of the planet's oxygen, and because of its unique nutritional properties and microscopic size, it is believed to penetrate the cellular level of the body, thereby enabling fast nutritional support to all the body's organs and systems. By strengthening the cells directly, phytoplankton's nutrients can help restore health and vitality in the entire body. Ultimately, cancer and other disorders occur when nutrients are missing on the cellular level. Since phytoplankton contains nearly all nutrients that exist on the planet, and delivery of these nutrients does not depend on the efficiency of the digestive system, this superfood may quickly provide whatever the body may be missing. For more information and testimonials, see www.ener-chi.com.

Other Useful Cancer Therapies

Dozens of other natural cancer therapies have helped millions of people regain their health, without aggressive medical intervention. Although this book's purpose is to reveal the true causes of cancer and how to address them, I also wish to acknowledge the great potential benefits these natural cancer remedies have. I have already described some of them in more detail, but this in no way diminishes the value of others. These include:

- Ayurveda's Pancha Karma treatment and herbal remedies
- Yoga
- Hydrazine Sulfate
- Antineoplaston therapy
- Acupuncture
- Bioelectric therapy
- Bioresonance therapy
- Royal Rife Machine therapy
- Gerson therapy
- Hoxsey therapy
- Therapies using Iscador (Mistletoe), Pau D'Arco, Chaparral,

Aloe Vera, Graviola
- Homeopathy
- The Coley Vaccine
- The Camphor Therapy of Gaston Naessens
- Burton's Immuno-augmentative therapy
- Livingston therapy
- Issels' Whole Body therapy
- Metabolic therapy by Hans Nieper, M.D.
- Live Cell therapy
- Chelation therapy
- Hyperthermia
- DMSO therapy
- The Cesium Chloride Protcol
- Oleander Treatment (oleander plant)
- Intravenous Hydrogen Peroxide
- IP6
- Dr. Simoncini's Baking Soda treatment
- Edgar Cayce's Castor Oil Packs
- Dr. Budwig Diet
- Dr. Clark's Parasite/Cancer treatments
- Moerman's Anti-Cancer Diet
- Red Clover Tea[56]
- Liquid Cellular Zeolites (www.mywaiora.com/500062)
- And more....

Alternative cancer therapies would be a lot more successful than they are if patients didn't use them as a last resort, that is, after all other approaches have failed. Unfortunately, almost every person diagnosed with cancer picks the orthodox medical approach. Most cancer patients believe that the doctor-prescribed

---

[56] Although red clover's anti-cancer effects are anecdotal, they are being confirmed as a traditional cancer remedy. Women with breast cancer were able to stop cancer growth by drinking red clover tea in place of water. Take one cup of clover herb and place it in one gallon of boiling water; allow it to seep for 20 minutes, strain and refrigerate. Drink 6-8 glasses (8 oz.) per day, at room temperature or warm.

orthodox treatments offer them a 40% chance of "beating that thing." However, the true likelihood of surviving the cancer, and more importantly, the cancer treatment, is actually less than 3%.[57] And there is no guarantee for those 3% who survive that they will not suffer from a new bout of cancer or a different, equally debilitating illness in the future.

The side-effects resulting from orthodox cancer therapy are so severe that those surviving cancer patients then choosing alternative cancer treatments are often disappointed that the new, natural treatments just "didn't work." The problem is that over 95% of cancer patients seeking help from natural cancer therapies have already been given up by orthodox medicine. In other words, the medical treatment has destroyed their body to a point that healing is very difficult to achieve. Their immune system is severely compromised, liver functions have been impaired, and the digestive system is too weak to make proper use of the food they eat. Unless a potent alternative therapy includes restoring these important parts and functions, the chances of it bringing about a complete cure are indeed slim. The true cure rate using natural approaches could exceed 90% if the body's key healing systems weren't severely damaged or destroyed by previously administered medical treatments. The less damage these treatments have caused, the stronger is the likelihood of recovery.

While I bring the above-listed alternative, natural approaches to your attention, I also wish to recommend that you don't lose sight of the true nature, origins, and progressive stages of cancer and general illness, as described in this and my other books, *The Amazing Liver and Gallbladder Flush* and *Timeless Secrets of Health and Rejuvenation.*

It is easy to become so overwhelmed by the physical appearance and reality of a cancerous tumor that you may impatiently focus on finding a "cure" and forsake attending to the ultimate, less obvious causes of cancer. The cancerous tumor

---

[57] This is the average 5-year survival rate for all medically treated cancers. It may be higher or lower, given the type of cancer. It excludes the millions of non-fatal skin cancers which the orthodox medical system conveniently includes in their statistical calculations to boost their success rate.

already is the body's attempt at curing the real cancer. The intention to combat cancer, even with such relatively natural methods as listed above, is similar to trying to enforce peace by waging a war. But we all know that this strategy rarely works. If you choose one or more of these methods, make certain you don't use them with the intention to kill something, especially a tumor. Any of these approaches may or may not be useful in supporting the body to heal, but you must never forget that, ultimately, the healing is done in the body and by the body, and is especially determined by what is going on in your heart and mind.

The intention behind your decision is more powerful than what you choose as your therapeutic tool. If fear motivates your decision making, you may be better off taking no action at all until you can face, embrace, and transform that fear into trust and confidence. Fear has a paralyzing effect and undermines the body's ability to heal. It is well known that the body cannot heal well when it is under stress. Stress hormones suppress digestive functions, eliminative functions, the immune system, and blood circulation to vital organs. Perceiving a cancer as a threat to your life makes it stressful. Perceiving it as a healing attempt by the body or a solution to an underlying unresolved conflict gives it meaning and purpose, and thus, it will not invoke a stress response.

Eventually, there will come a time when you no longer perceive the lump in your chest or the tumor in your colon or brain as a problem, but as an essential part of the solution to a deeper unresolved issue in your life that may have been buried so deep inside you that you weren't even aware of it. Cancer can bring to the surface what was concealed for a long time and allow you to make peace with it, accept it, and even embrace it. A lump in the breast or a tumor in the brain is merely a manifestation of resistance—resistance against yourself, against others, or against situations and circumstances. When it no longer matters to you whether a lump is getting bigger or smaller, you will practically stop feeding it with your energies.

Healing occurs when there is no more need to fix what you believe is broken. The need to fix it still reflects an incomplete perception or acceptance of yourself, based on the fear of not

204

being good enough, strong enough, or deserving enough. The lump or tumor helps you to be in touch with that insecurity and vulnerability, and transform these into courage and confidence. It challenges you to live happily and enjoy your life even with the cancer. When you have risen to meet this challenge, which is achieved through simple acceptance of its deeper meaning and purpose, the need for the cancer will be gone along with the insecurity.

To repeat, the lump or tumor is not the problem. What is important is how you react to it. If you could live with it comfortably and without much concern or wanting to kill it off, you are close to experiencing a spontaneous remission. The size of a tumor is quite irrelevant. In fact, it can increase in size when it is healing, due to increased lymphocyte activity. And then it may vanish quickly. I once saw an orange-size bladder tumor displayed live on an ultrasound screen completely disintegrate and disappear within 15 seconds. Know that the body is always on your side, and never against you, however bad the situation may appear to be. In fact, nothing in your life is ever against you, even pain is a way of breaking your resistance to what is actually good for you, but you cannot yet see it that way. You can learn from everything that happens to you, including cancer.

In any case, it is far more important to identify and address whatever prevents the body from healing, or rather, to supply whatever helps it to feel whole and vital, than to fix the symptomatic appearance of a cancer.

Summary and Concluding Remarks:
Healing the Ultimate Cause

My intention in writing this book was to offer an alternative view of what cancer is, one that reflects the intelligence and purpose of nature's laws. Important and commonsense reasons govern the constructive forces of natural law; the same is true of natural law's destructive forces. If it were otherwise, growth would not occur, and the universe as we know it would have vanished long ago. Everything has meaning, regardless how meaningless it may appear to be. An apple can only grow (constructive force of natural law) after the blossom that precedes it has been destroyed (destructive force of natural law). **He who finds purpose and meaning in the occurrence of a cancer will also find the way to cure it.** This is the promise of this book. It is a matter of tracing a cancer back to its origins—the various layers of preceding causes and effects.

The ultimate cause of cancer is fear—fear of not being good enough, fear of loss, fear of being hurt, fear of hurting others, fear of loving, fear of not loving enough, fear of disappointment, fear of success, fear of failure, fear of dying, fear of food, fear of being disappointed, and fear of life and existence. Each of these fears is but an offspring of the fear of the unknown.

The fear of the unknown is not a tangible thing that you can just get rid of by deciding to. More often than not, you manifest what you are afraid of. Negative expectations are self-fulfilling prophecies. When these prophecies or expectations become fulfilled, it may give you the idea that they would have occurred anyway, as if you had no choice. Yet, you always have a choice. You are never a victim of anything or anyone, even it feels that way, which is the point. You can only be a victim when you feel like one. Although we often create what we fear through subconscious programming, we can just as easily change the program and create what we love.

To heal cancer, you must first know deep within yourself that your body does not have the ability to do you any harm. Therefore, you need not be afraid of it. Through the eyes of acceptance, you will be capable of seeing any negative situation in life, such as the occurrence of a cancerous tumor, in a positive light.[58] This inner transformation of perspective immediately dispels the fear of the unknown. Once you accept an injury or an illness as something that can benefit you, e.g. strengthen you in an area of your life where you have felt weak, incompetent, or anxious before, you will start connecting with it. This connection

---

[58] To develop this ability, see *Lifting the Veil of Duality – Your Guide to Living without Judgment.*

with the "problem" then allows your energy and emotion to flow into it and release the emotional barriers to spontaneous healing.

As mentioned before, healing cannot occur when the life force is absent. Life force is unavailable when you are "absent," when you separate yourself from the body and its predicament or illness. You do this when you perceive or imagine it to be turning against you, or even trying to kill you. Whenever you are afraid of the body, you will try either to protect yourself from it or fight against it. In either case, this strong feeling of being alienated from the body sucks the life force out of every cell. Your cells go into protection or fighting mode, commonly known as the fight or flight response. Hence, their life force energy is wasted, which prevents them from growing, healing, and regenerating themselves.

Tumors of any kind are direct manifestations of fear. Fear is synonymous with separation and defensiveness. Cancer cells do not like what they have become, but your resistance to them keeps them in that state. They heal spontaneously when your resistance disappears and you are able to replace this attitude with one of acceptance and, yes, love. When you consciously accept/embrace what or whom you resist in your life (whom or what you resist is merely a mirror image of yourself[59]), you will not only lose the fear, but also the body's cells can return to their natural, balanced growth mode. Balanced growth always results in homeostasis or health. Cleansing, pampering, and nourishing the body are acts of accepting responsibility for what is happening to you, and they return to you true ownership of your body. Taking your power back where it belongs and letting go of external crutches, like suppressive drugs, aggressive treatments, surgery, etc., are essential for healing yourself, i.e. your body, mind, and emotions.

The power of thoughts, feelings, and emotions is many times stronger than any physical influence can be. Yes, you may have a tumor in your breast or in your brain, but you are still more

---

[59] For details see *Lifting the Veil of Duality—Your Guide to Living Without Judgment.*

powerful and influential than the tumor is. In fact, your own energy of fear or resistance has created it and sustains it. In the same way you feed the tumor, your energy of love and acceptance can crumble its foundation and undo it. Do not fall into the trap of believing the body is causing you problems that you cannot heal. The theory that cancer is a life-threatening disease that has a separate power or agenda other than your own is just an acquired belief, and yet beliefs shape reality. The body does not have the power to cause you any ailments; on the contrary, it is ever vigilant to resolve them in the best possible way it can, circumstances permitting.

You are the creator of your circumstances. It is for you to decide every morning when you wake up whether to spend the day recounting the difficulties you have with the parts of your body that no longer work properly, or to be thankful for the ones that do work. The same applies to every other problem in your life. It is within your power to choose between watering the roots of a withering plant or lamenting over its falling leaves.

You can do much in terms of self-healing that you may never have thought of before. Show your body that you are not afraid of it. Place both hands over your dis-eased organ or gland. Thank the cancer cells for the precious work they have done for you. Give thanks to all the cells that have managed to keep you alive, despite the toxins and congestion that have impeded their work. Infuse them with the life force that is inside you by appreciating them and accepting them back into your awareness and presence. The DNA of your cells can hear you just as well as you can hear someone speaking to you, as Russian DNA research has demonstrated. The body primarily runs by vibration. Expressing gratitude to the cells of your body and for the challenges and blessings life presents you with, acts as one of the most powerful vibrations you can produce. The energy of "thank you" actually reconnects you with whatever you have separated yourself from. This makes gratitude the major secret and prerequisite for healing to occur.

With a renewed, more loving, and compassionate attitude toward your cancer cells—remember, they are still your body's cells—you can truly start healing the physical and non-physical causes of cancer. You, yourself, will become living proof that **cancer is not a disease.**

WISHING YOU PERFECT HEALTH, ABUNDANCE AND HAPPINESS !

Andreas Moritz

Other Books, Products, and Services by the Author

The Amazing Liver & Gallbladder Flush
A Powerful Do-It-Yourself Tool to Optimize Your Health and Wellbeing

In this revised edition of his best selling book, *The Amazing Liver Cleanse,* Andreas Moritz addresses the most common but rarely recognized cause of illness—gallstones congesting the liver. Although those who suffer an excruciatingly painful gallbladder attack are clearly aware of the stones congesting this vital organ, few people realize that hundreds if not thousands of gallstones (mainly clumps of hardened bile) have accumulated in their liver, often causing no pain or symptoms for decades. Most adults living in the industrialized world, and especially those suffering a chronic illness such as heart disease, arthritis, MS, cancer, or diabetes, have gallstones blocking the bile ducts of their liver. Furthermore, 20 million Americans suffer from gallbladder attacks every year. In many cases, treatment consists merely of removing the gallbladder, at the cost of $5 billion a year. This purely symptom-oriented approach, however, does not eliminate the cause of the illness, and in many cases, sets the stage for even more serious conditions.

This book provides a thorough understanding of what causes gallstones in both the liver and gallbladder and explains why these stones can be held responsible for the most common diseases so prevalent in the world today. It provides the reader with the knowledge needed to recognize the stones and gives the necessary, do-it-yourself instructions to remove them painlessly in the comfort of one's own home. The book also shares practical guidelines on how to prevent new gallstones from forming. The widespread success of *The Amazing Liver & Gallbladder Flush* stands as a testimony to the strength and effectiveness of the cleanse itself. This powerful yet simple cleanse has led to extraordinary improvements in health and wellness among thousands of people who have already given themselves the precious gift of a strong, clean, revitalized liver.

Timeless Secrets of
Health and Rejuvenation
Breakthrough Medicine for the 21st Century
(550 pages, 8 ½ x 11 inches)

This book meets the increasing demand for a clear and comprehensive guide that can helps people to become self-sufficient regarding their health and wellbeing. It answers some of the most pressing questions of our time: How does illness arise? Who heals, and who doesn't? Are we destined to be sick? What causes aging? Is it reversible? What are the major causes of disease, and how can we eliminate them? What simple and effective practices can I incorporate into my daily routine that will dramatically improve my health?

Topics include: The placebo effect and the mind/body mystery; the laws of illness and health; the four most common risk factors for disease; digestive disorders and their effects on the rest of the body; the wonders of our biological rhythms and how to restore them if disrupted; how to create a life of balance; why to choose a vegetarian diet; cleansing the liver, gallbladder, kidneys, and colon; removing allergies; giving up smoking, naturally; using sunlight as medicine; the "new" causes of heart disease, cancer, diabetes, and AIDS; and a scrutinizing look at antibiotics, blood transfusions, ultrasound scans, and immunization programs.

Timeless Secrets of Health and Rejuvenation sheds light on all major issues of healthcare and reveals that most medical treatments, including surgery, blood transfusions, and pharmaceutical drugs, are avoidable when certain key functions in the body are restored through the natural methods described in the book. The reader also learns about the potential dangers of medical diagnosis and treatment, as well as the reasons vitamin

212

supplements, "health foods," low-fat products, "wholesome" breakfast cereals, diet foods, and diet programs may have contributed to the current health crisis rather than helped to resolve it. The book includes a complete program of healthcare, which is primarily based on the ancient medical system of Ayurveda and the vast amount of experience Andreas Moritz has gained in the field of health restoration during the past 30 years.

Lifting the Veil of Duality
Your Guide to Living Without Judgment

"Do you know that there is a place inside you – hidden beneath the appearance of thoughts, feelings, and emotions – that does not know the difference between good and evil, right and wrong, light and dark? From that place you embrace the opposite values of life as *One*. In this sacred place you are at peace with yourself and at peace with your world." - *Andreas Moritz*

In *Lifting the Veil of Duality,* Andreas Moritz poignantly exposes the illusion of duality. He outlines a simple way to remove every limitation that you have imposed upon yourself during the course of living in the realm of duality. You will be prompted to see yourself and the world through a new lens – the lens of clarity, discernment, and non-judgment. You will also discover that mistakes, accidents, coincidences, negativity, deception, injustice, wars, crime, and terrorism all have a deeper purpose and meaning in the larger scheme of things. So naturally, much of what you will read may conflict with the beliefs you currently hold. Yet you are not asked to change your beliefs or opinions. Instead, you are asked to have *an open mind,* for only an open mind can enjoy freedom from judgment.

Our personal views and worldviews are currently challenged by a crisis of identity. Some are being shattered altogether. The collapse of our current world order forces humanity to deal with the most basic issues of existence. You can no longer avoid taking responsibility for the things that happen to you. When you *do* accept responsibility, you also empower and heal yourself.

Lifting the Veil of Duality shows you how you create or

213

subdue your ability to fulfill your desires. Furthermore, you will find intriguing explanations about the mystery of time, the truth and illusion of reincarnation, the oftentimes misunderstood value of prayer, what makes relationships work, and why so often they don't. Find out why injustice is an illusion that has managed to haunt us throughout the ages. Learn about our original separation from the Source of life and what this means with regard to the current waves of instability and fear so many of us are experiencing.

Discover how to identify the angels living amongst us and why we all have light-bodies. You will have the opportunity to find the ultimate God within you and discover why a God seen as separate from yourself keeps you from being in your Divine Power and happiness. In addition, you can find out how to heal yourself at a moment's notice. Read all about the "New Medicine" and the destiny of the old medicine, the old economy, the old religion, and the old world.

It's Time to Come Alive!
Start Using the Amazing Healing Powers of Your Body, Mind, and Spirit Today!

In this book, the author brings to light man's deep inner need for spiritual wisdom in life and helps the reader develop a new sense of reality that is based on love, power, and compassion. He describes our relationship with the natural world in detail and discusses how we can harness its tremendous powers for our personal and humanity's benefit. *It's Time to Come Alive* challenges some of our most commonly held beliefs and offers a way out of the emotional restrictions and physical limitations we have created in our lives.

Topics include: What shapes our destiny; using the power of intention; secrets of defying the aging process; doubting – the cause of failure; opening the heart; material wealth and spiritual wealth; fatigue – the major cause of stress; methods of emotional transformation; techniques of primordial healing; how to increase the health of the five senses; developing spiritual wisdom; the

214

major causes of today's earth changes; entry into the new world; 12 gateways to heaven on earth; and many more.

Simple Steps to Total Health!
Andreas Moritz with co-author John Hornecker

By nature, your physical body is designed to be healthy and vital throughout life. Unhealthy eating habits and lifestyle choices, however, lead to numerous health conditions that prevent you from enjoying life to the fullest. In *Simple Steps to Total Health*, the authors bring to light the most common cause of disease, which is the build-up of toxins and residues from improperly digested foods that inhibit various organs and systems from performing their normal functions. This guidebook for total health provides you with simple but highly effective approaches for internal cleansing, hydration, nutrition, and living habits.

The book's three parts cover the essentials of total health – Good Internal Hygiene, Healthy Nutrition, and Balanced Lifestyle. Learn about the most common disease-causing foods, dietary habits and influences responsible for the occurrence of chronic illnesses, including those affecting the blood vessels, heart, liver, intestinal organs, lungs, kidneys, joints, bones, nervous system, and sense organs.

To be able to live a healthy life, you must align your internal biological rhythms with the larger rhythms of nature. Find out more about this and many other important topics in *Simple Steps to Total Health*. This is a "must-have" book for anyone who is interested in using a natural, drug-free approach to restore total health.

Heart Disease No More!
Make Peace with Your Heart
and Heal Yourself
(Excerpted from Timeless Secrets of Health and Rejuvenation)

Less than one hundred years ago, heart disease was an

extremely rare illness. Today it kills more people in the developed world than all other causes of death combined. Despite the vast quantity of financial resources spent on finding a cure for heart disease, the current medical approaches remain mainly symptom-oriented and do not address the underlying causes.

Even worse, overwhelming evidence shows that the treatment of heart disease or its presumed precursors, such as high blood pressure, hardening of the arteries, and high cholesterol, not only prevents a real cure, but also can easily lead to chronic heart failure. The patient's heart may still beat, but not strongly enough for him to feel vital and alive.

Without removing the underlying causes of heart disease and its precursors, the average person has little, if any, protection against it. Heart attacks can strike whether you have undergone a coronary bypass or had stents placed inside your arteries. According to research, these procedures fail to prevent heart attacks and do nothing to reduce mortality rates.

Heart Disease No More, excerpted from the author's bestselling book, *Timeless Secrets of Health and Rejuvenation*, puts the responsibility for healing where it belongs, on the heart, mind, and body of each individual. It provides the reader with practical insights about the development and causes of heart disease. Even better, it explains simple steps you can take to prevent and reverse heart disease for good, regardless of a possible genetic predisposition.

Diabetes--No More!
Discover and Heal Its True Causes
(Excerpted from Timeless Secrets of
Health and Rejuvenation)

According to this bestselling author, diabetes is not a disease; in the vast majority of cases, it is a complex mechanism of protection or survival that the body chooses to avoid the possibly fatal consequences of an unhealthful diet and lifestyle.

Despite the body's ceaseless self-preservation efforts (which we call diseases), millions of people suffer or die unnecessarily from these consequences. The imbalanced blood sugar level in diabetes is but a symptom of illness, not the illness itself. By developing diabetes, the body is neither doing something wrong, nor is it trying to commit suicide. The current diabetes epidemic is man-made, or rather, factory-made, and, therefore, can be halted and reversed through simple but effective changes in diet and lifestyle. *Diabetes—No More* provides you with essential information on the various causes of diabetes and how anyone can avoid them.

To stop the diabetes epidemic you need to create the right circumstances that allow your body to heal. Just as there is a mechanism to become diabetic, there is also a mechanism to reverse it. Find out how!

This book was excerpted from the bestselling book, *Timeless Secrets of Health and Rejuvenation.*

Ending The AIDS Myth
It's Time to Heal the TRUE Causes!
(Excerpted from Timeless Secrets of Health and Rejuvenation)

Contrary to common belief, no scientific evidence exists to this day to prove that AIDS is a contagious disease. The current AIDS theory falls short in predicting the kind of AIDS disease an infected person may be manifesting, and no accurate system is in place to determine how long it will take for the disease to develop. In addition, the current HIV/AIDS theory contains no reliable information that can help identify those who are at risk for developing AIDS.

On the other hand, published research actually proves that HIV only spreads heterosexually in extremely rare cases and cannot be responsible for an epidemic that involves millions of AIDS victims around the world. Furthermore, it is an established fact that the retrovirus HIV, which is composed of human gene fragments, is incapable of destroying human cells. However, cell destruction is the main characteristic of every AIDS disease.

Even the principal discoverer of HIV, Luc Montagnier, no

217

longer believes that HIV is solely responsible for causing AIDS. In fact, he showed that HIV alone could not cause AIDS. Increasing evidence indicates that AIDS may be a toxicity syndrome or metabolic disorder that is caused by immunity risk factors, including heroin, sex-enhancement drugs, antibiotics, commonly prescribed AIDS drugs, rectal intercourse, starvation, malnutrition, and dehydration.

Dozens of prominent scientists working at the forefront of AIDS research now openly question the virus hypothesis of AIDS. Find out why! *Ending the AIDS Myth* also shows you what really causes the shutdown of the immune system and what you can do to avoid this.

All books are available paperback and as electronic books through the Ener-Chi Wellness Center

Website: http://www.ener-chi.com
Email: support@ener-chi.com

Toll free 1(866) 258-4006 (USA)
Local: 1(709) 570-7401 (Canada)

Telephone Consultations

For a Personal Telephone Consultation with Andreas Moritz, please:

1. Call or send an email with your name, phone number, address, digital picture (if you have one) of your face, and any other relevant information to:

E-mail: andmor@ener-chi.com

Telephone: 1 (864) 895-6285 (USA)

2. Set up an appointment for the length of time you choose to spend with him. A comprehensive consultation lasts two hours or more. Shorter consultations deal with all the questions you may have and any information that is relevant to your specific health issue(s). **For current fees please visit the consultation page at:** http://www.ener-chi.com

To order Books, Ener-Chi Art pictures and Ionized Stones
please contact:

Ener-Chi Wellness Center, LLC

Website: http://www.ener-chi.com
Toll free: 1 (866) 258-4006 (USA)
Local: 1 (709) 570-7401 (Canada)

ABOUT THE AUTHOR

Andreas Moritz is a medical intuitive; a practitioner of Ayurveda, iridology, shiatsu, and vibrational medicine; a writer; and an artist. Born in southwest Germany in 1954, Moritz had to deal with several severe illnesses from an early age, which compelled him to study diet, nutrition, and various methods of natural healing while still a child.

By the age of 20, he had completed his training in both iridology—the diagnostic science of eye interpretation—and dietetics. In 1981, he began studying Ayurvedic medicine in India and finished his training as a qualified practitioner of Ayurveda in New Zealand in 1991. Rather than being satisfied with merely treating the symptoms of illness, Moritz has dedicated his life's work to understanding and treating the root causes of illness. Because of this holistic approach, he has had great success with cases of terminal disease where conventional methods of healing proved futile.

Since 1988, he has practiced the Japanese healing art of shiatsu, which has given him insights into the energy system of the body. In addition, he devoted eight years of research into consciousness and its important role in the field of mind/body medicine.

Andreas Moritz is also the author of *Timeless Secrets of Health and Rejuvenation, The Amazing Liver and Gallbladder Flush, Lifting the Veil of Duality, It's Time to Come Alive, Heart Disease No More, Simple Steps to Total Health, Diabetes—No More, Ending the AIDS Myth* and *Heal Yourself with Sunlight.*

During his extensive travels throughout the world, he has consulted with heads of state and members of government in Europe, Asia, and Africa, and has lectured widely on the subjects of health, mind/body medicine, and spirituality. His popular *Timeless Secrets of Health and Rejuvenation* workshops assist people in taking responsibility for their own health and wellbeing. Moritz has a free forum, "Ask Andreas Moritz," on the large health website curezone.com (five million readers and increasing). Although he recently stopped writing for the forum, it contains an extensive archive of his answers to thousands of questions on a variety of health topics.

Since taking up residence in the United States in 1998, Moritz has been involved in developing a new and innovative system of healing—called *Ener-Chi Art*—that targets the root causes of many chronic illnesses. Ener-Chi Art consists of a series of light ray-encoded oil paintings that can instantly restore vital energy flow (Chi) in the organs and systems of the body. Moritz is also the founder of *Sacred Santémony—Divine Chanting for Every Occasion,* a powerful system of specially generated frequencies of sound that can transform deep-seated fears, allergies, traumas, and mental or emotional blocks into useful opportunities for growth and inspiration within a matter of moments.

INDEX

x, 197
Biochemical Journal, 83
Biofeedback, 178
Biopsy, 139, 140
Black cohosh, 174
Blood, 17, 19, 34, 35, 43, 49, 51, 52,
    54, 55, 56, 57, 58, 59, 62, 64, 65,
    68, 71, 72, 73, 112, 115, 116, 132,
    134, 137, 138, 140, 144, 158, 160,
    188, 189, 193, 212, 215, 216, 217
    thickened, 55
Blood transfusions, 165
Blood vessel walls begin to thicken,
    52
Blood, 54, 55
Blood-thickening, 54, 55, 158
Blood-thickening agent, 54
Bras
    impair proper lymph flow, 147
Brassica vegetables, 174
Breast cancer, 1, 14, 15, 21, 27, 60,
    96, 99, 104, 105, 106, 111, 112,
    125, 128, 147, 148, 150, 154, 155,
    161, 163, 165, 167, 168, 169, 170,
    174, 176, 180, 182, 187, 192, 202
Breast Cancer, 125, 148, 150, 154,
    187
Breast Cancers
    DCIS, 15
Brine, 88
British Journal of Urology
    International, 141
Burdock Root, 195

C

Cadaverines, 65
Caffeine, 77, 102, 159, 160
Calcium & Cancer, 140
Canadian Medical Association
    Journal, 109
Cancer,
    *& physical, emotional and spiritual
        issues*, xiv
    & poor self-image, xiii
    a killer disease?, 3
    a survival mechanism, 11
    all Cancers can be survived, 5
    *behind the mask of its physical
        symptoms*, xiii

*Behind the mask of its physical
    symptoms.*, xiii
Causes, xi, xii, xiv, xv, 39, 44, 46,
    53, 103, 161, 172, 178, 201,
    203, 209
Cellular balance, 10
Complex survival response, xi
*Constant conflicts, guilt and shame
    are some of the examples of
    events that can lead to Cancer*,
    xiii
Dealing with unresolved conflicts,
    xiv
Defective genes, 9
*Important questions to address by
    cancer sufferers*, xi
Influence of the external
    environment on cells, 10
Its manifestation just from
    believing you have it, 16
Medical cancer therapy a
    treatment?, 15
Not a disease, 3
Not a killer, xiii
Ovarian, 54
Survival rates, 27
*The result of many crises of
    toxicity,* 129
Cancer, a powerful healer, ix, 122
Cancer, a response to rejection, ix,
    117
Cancer, a survival mechanism, 11
Cancer and heart disease, viii, 56, 58
Cancer cell definition, 33, 40
Cancer cells have no ability to kill
    anything, 33
Cancer, guilt and shame, 120
Cancer has never killed a person, 32
Cancer is not loving yourself, ix
Cancer is on our side, xi
Cancer Journal, 178
Cancer, result of many crises of
    toxicity, 129
Cancer resurrects numbed, suppressed
    or congested areas, 46
Cancer statistics
    expected number of victims, 1
Cancer therapy
    scientific?, 15
Cancer treatments

Food ddditives
their effect on genes, 10
Food products & nutritional value, 74
Formaldehyde, 145, 162
Fred Hutchinson Cancer Research
Center, 140
Free radicals, 39, 40, 54, 60, 61, 95,
96, 196
French fries, 60, 74, 80, 82, 153
Fried chicken, 60
Fructose and sucrose, 165
Fungi, 34, 37, 67, 193, 199, 200

G

Gastrointestinal problems, xv, 25, 100,
107, 134, 138, 183, 184
Gene, 53, 41
Genes, vii, xiii, 8, 9, 11, 16, 32, 40,
41, 42, 45, 57, 115, 136, 137
it's purpose, 12
not to blame, xiii
their true purpose, 12
Genetic blueprints
cannot cause disease, 9
Genetic design, xii, 42
Genetic mutation, 33, 35, 42, 134,
136, 184
a normal survival response, 11
Germs don't cause cancer, vii, 36
Ginger, 175, 176
Gingerol, 176
Ginseng, 175
Glucose, 42, 43, 50, 51, 52, 56, 60, 64,
130, 136, 137, 177, 198
Glycemic index, 177
Goji juice, 175
Grape seed, 175
Graviola, x, 175, 191, 192, 193, 202
Green tea, 175
Growth hormones
& cancer, 163
Guilt, xiii, 113, 120, 122, 124, 126
unjustified and unnecessary, 122
Gum Disease
& cancer, viii, 88

H

Hair dye, 161

Hair follicles
inflammation of cells, xv
Hardening of the arteries, 55, 59, 216
Harvard Medical School, 62
Heal what is only yours to heal, 105
Healing, vi, vii, x, xi, xiv, 3, 5, 7, 21,
22, 23, 36, 40, 45, 80, 116, 124,
133, 143, 145, 188, 189, 190, 192,
204, 205, 207, 208, 214, 216
Healing cancer versus fighting it, vii,
3
Healing crisis, 86, 143, 145, 146, 172,
192
Healing response, 29, 36, 40, 110
Healing the causes of cancer must
include restoring one's physical,
emotional and spiritual well-being,
xiv
Hemoglobin, 92
Hemorrhage, 106, 143
Herbs, 142, 174, 175, 177, 178, 197
*list of herbs with anti-cancer
properties*, 174
positive effects of herbs, 174
Herceptin, 106
Heroin, 77, 218
HIV, 104, 194, 217
Hodgkin's disease, 14, 71, 117
Homeostasis, 47, 74, 207
Hope
there is no false hope, 4
HRT, 104
Human body, the most complex
system in the universe, 133
Human genome, 12
Human papillomavirus (HPV), 38
Hydrochloric acid, 54, 104
Hydrogenated vegetable oils, 62
Hydroxide, 145
Hypnosis, 178

I

Immune system, 48, 92, 112, 134,
138, 144, 145, 146, 150
Immune systems, 13, 42, 146
compromised, effect of
chemotherapy, 13
Immunity, 37, 111, 128, 145, 146, 218
Immunization programs, 145, 146,

212
Infection, 19, 35, 36, 37, 38, 49, 88,
  106, 135, 137, 139, 197
  prevents cancer, 35
Infections prevented or suppressed, 40
Infrared Thermal Imaging
  to detect breast cancer, 169
Innate healing ability, 20
Interferon, 10, 37
Interleukin II, 6, 10
  the body's anti-cancer drug, 6
International Journal of Cancer, 83,
  142
International Journal of Toxicology,
  87
Intestines, 115
  large intestine, 115
Intrahepatic stones, 55, 72, 112, 118
Ionizing radiation, 166
Iridology, 118

J

Johns Hopkins University, 72, 186
Joints, 14, 70, 112, 189, 196, 198, 215
Junk foods, 2, 151

K

Kidney cancer, 3, 49, 143, 173
Kidneys, xv, 3, 40, 54, 98, 108, 109,
  150, 159, 161, 164, 173, 192, 212,
  215
Killer disease, 5
Killing the cancer implies we kill the
  patient, 130

L

Lactic acid, 42, 57, 132, 136, 137, 174
LDL cholesterol, 59
Legumes
  Enzyme inhibitors, 150
Leukemia, 14, 88, 162, 166
Leukemia
  caused by chemotherapy, 14
Life force (Chi), 33, 188, 189, 207,
  208
Life-long dependency on doctors, 19
List of other Cancer therapies, 201

Liver, iii, viii, 40, 51, 54, 55, 65, 71,
  72, 73, 74, 104, 112, 115, 116, 118,
  120, 137, 138, 142, 144, 161, 173,
  188, 189, 193, 203, 211, 212, 215,
  220
  & control over growth/functioning
    of cells in the body, 73
Liver cancer, 53, 79, 104
Liver cleanse
  gallstones, 120, 138
Liver congestion and cancer, heart
  disease and other chronic illnesses,
  73
Louis Pasteur, 35
Love, 23, 113, 118, 119, 120, 121,
  126, 127, 172, 173, 206, 207, 208,
  214
Lumps, 70
Lung cancer, 1, 15, 27, 53, 88, 107
Lungs, xv, 51, 58, 70, 144, 166, 215
Lupus, 104, 194, 195
Lymph cancer, 117
Lymphatic congestion, 65, 67, 70, 71,
  170, 184
  & liver congestion, 71
  illness caused by, 70
Lymphatic system, 35, 36, 40, 57, 64,
  65, 67, 68, 119, 188, 199
  key functions, 65
Lymphedema, 67, 68, 69
Lymphoma, 14, 18, 71, 117, 166, 171

M

Maintaining regular meal times, x, 183
Malignant tumors, xi, 14, 68, 144
Mammogram, 155, 168
Mammography, 155, 167, 168, 169,
  170
Manufactured foods, 75, 77, 80, 82, 93
Many people have cancer in their
  body and will never know about it,
  133
Margarine, 61, 62, 81
Marjoram, 175
Massage, 178
Mastectomy, 111
Mayo Clinic, 13, 99
Meal times
  & healing cancer, x, 183

227

Parkinson's disease, 52
Parsley, 175
Pau D 'Arco, 175
Paxil, 104
Permixon, 141
Pesticides and other chemical toxins,
    160
Pharmaceutical companies, 12, 24, 28,
    29
Pharmaceutical drugs cause cancer,
    103
Phlegm, 138
Physician-caused fatalities, 27
Phytoestrogens, 150, 151
Pineal gland, 180, 181
Placebo effect, 12, 16, 212
Placebo effect works both ways, 16
Plaque, 39, 58, 59, 89, 90
Platelets, 52, 62, 101
Pleomorphism, 34
Pneumonia, 101, 143, 144, 194
Polio shots, 146
Polyunsaturated fats, 60, 61
    & risk of breast cancer, 60
    & sunlight, 61
Power of thoughts, feelings, and
    emotions, 207
Prednisone, cortisone, and other
    steroids, 104
Prescription drugs, 22, 109, 141
Prognosis, 3, 4, 5
Prostate, 1, 6, 54, 70, 88, 99, 100, 125,
    132, 139, 140, 141, 142, 161, 163,
    165, 175, 192
Prostate biopsy, 139
Prostate cancer
    only 1 percent die, 6
Prostate cancer, ix, 139
Protein, viii, 9, 51, 52, 54, 55, 56, 58,
    59, 60, 67, 78, 81, 104, 108, 115,
    125, 134, 136, 146, 149, 150, 152,
    185, 186
Protein (animal), 53, 54, 60, 67, 93,
    108, 115, 185, 186
Protein foods most acid forming, 55
Protein-cancer connection, 52
Protits, 34
PSA (prostate-specific-antigen), 139
PSA test
    to detect prostate cancer, 139, 140

Puberty and breast cancer link, ix, 148
Purple corn, 82
Purpose of our existence, 127
Putrescines, 65
PVC shower-curtains, 162

R

Radiation, xii, xv, 3, 7, 13, 17, 21, 23,
    24, 26, 27, 29, 38, 41, 76, 79, 80,
    84, 85, 86, 87, 88, 93, 96, 111, 118,
    120, 121, 130, 156, 160, 166, 167,
    168, 169, 171, 172, 178, 191
Radiolytics
    chemicals in microwaved foods,
        75, 155
Red blood cell, 30, 72, 92, 150, 166,
    200
Red Clover, 196, 202
Red Meat, 53, 82, 164, 186
Remission, 3, 4, 5, 13, 30, 36, 38, 80,
    116, 120, 130, 133, 134, 139, 171,
    172, 173, 205
Removal of symptoms once the causes
    are no longer present, 5
Repressed feelings, 114
Resentment, xiii, 2, 86, 122
Restoring Chi – the life force, x, 188
Rosemary, 175

S

Sacred Santémony, iii, x, 190, 191,
    221
Sage, 176
Saliva, 71
Sanguinary
    & gum disease, 89
Sarcoma, 76, 156
Saw palmetto, 141
Scavengers, 40
Scientific research, 11
Self healing
    *is about taking full responsibility of
        your body*, 5
Self respect, xiii
Self-destruction is not the theme of
    any cell, 33
Self-empowerment, 19
Septic shock, 43

NOTES

NOTES

NOTES